On Writing, Reading, and Dyslexia

SEMMELWEIS LECTURE, SPONSORED BY THE AMERICAN-
HUNGARIAN MEDICAL ASSOCIATION, NOVEMBER, 1968

ARTHUR LINKSZ, M.D.

*Clinical Professor of Ophthalmology, New York Medical College;
Consulting Surgeon, Manhattan Eye, Ear and Throat Hospital,
New York, New York*

GRUNE & STRATTON

New York — London

Library of Congress Cataloging in Publication Data
Linksz, Arthur.
    On writing, reading, and dyslexia.
    (Semmelweis lecture, 1968)
    Bibliography: p.
    1. English language — Study and teaching (Elementary)
2. Reading disability. 3. Dyslexia. 4. Left-
and right-handedness. I. Title. II. Series. [DMLN: 1. Dyslexia.
2. Reading. 3. Writing. WL340 L7560 1973]
LB1576.L54   428′.4   73-9978
ISBN 0-8089-0789-1

© 1973 by Grune & Stratton, Inc.

Grune & Stratton, Inc.
111 Fifth Avenue
New York, New York 10003

Library of Congress Catalog Card Number 73-9978
International Standard Book Number 0-8089-0789-1
Printed in the United States of America

CONTENTS

Also by Dr. Linksz

An Essay on Color Vision and Clinical Color Vision Tests, 1964
Physiology of the Eye: Volume I, Optics, 1950
Physiology of the Eye: Volume II, Vision, 1952

PREFACE

Although the problems of the poor reader have interested and intrigued me for many years, incentive to deal with the subject in an orderly fashion came with the invitation of my friends in the American-Hungarian Medical Association to deliver the annual Semmelweis lecture for the year 1968. I want to thank the president and members of the association for a great and most cherished honor.

I must say the lecture was well received, and several of my confreres encouraged me to publish it. As the subtitle of this volume indicates, this is an enlarged, quite enlarged, version of that speech.

I wish I could have added another subtitle — something like, *"A thirty-years' love affair of an immigrant with the English language."* It is comparable only to a convert's zeal for his adopted religion, this affection of mine for the English language. English spelling has been called so many bad names: "impossible," "unlearnable," "illogical," even "awful"; it behooves a hyphenated American to point out the beauty, the refined logic, the subtleties, in the spelling and in the structuring of English words. A considerable part of this book will be devoted to this — teaching English spelling with love.

I have also, and for many years, been interested in the history of writing, especially its kinetics, in the role of righthandedness in the ultimate evolution of Greco-Latin alphabets, and the problems inevitably met by the lefthander. Some of my best friends are lefthanders, and I must thank them for sharing their problems and their insights with me.

A chapter of this book is devoted to writing kinetics, to the vectors of writing, or more accurately, the vectors that form individual letters. Most of the sample letters to be discussed are Latin or Hebrew. I had the good fortune to meet a young Chinese-American ophthalmologist in San Francisco. With his help I gained some insight into the kinetics, the vectorial structure, of Chinese ideographic writing. Heartfelt thanks are due to this young colleague, Dr. Guy Wong.

Several friends and colleagues read my manuscript and made valuable suggestions. I want to offer them my thanks. But there is one among them, *Mr. Harry J. Groblewski* of Topsfield, Massachusetts, a dedicated educator, teacher, headmaster, school administrator, to whom I owe special tribute. Harry, my dear, very dear friend, spent endless hours reading and rereading my manuscript with me — discussing details, correcting errors, suggesting avenues, clarifying ambiguities, helping to add structure to what in its first transcripts was just a shapeless mass.

It is an old Latin saying that one learns best and most by teaching. An invitation in the fall of 1969 by Dr. Arthur Jampolsky, director of the Smith-Kettlewell Institute of Visual Sciences in San Francisco, to conduct a seminar on the subject of dyslexia made it possible for me further to organize my thoughts and their presentation. I think I profited more from these discussions than my listeners did — I found so many hazy items clarified. Here, again, thanks are due.

Special thanks go to my older son, Jim, for preparing most of the drawings and diagrams in the book. My love, affection, and thanks are due to my wife, Magda, and my two sons, Jim and David (to all of whom this volume is dedicated). Also apologies — I spent so much time writing books that I had little time to go with my sons to baseball games. They told me once that they will never forget this. Perhaps now they will forgive.

Arthur Linksz, M.D.

Consensus and History — Some Clinical Experiences With Poor Readers

Before I begin to elaborate on my topic, let me make two introductory remarks. The first will appear to be only loosely connected with what I am about to discuss. Still, I hope you will find it, if not pertinent, at least interesting.[1]

All of you who honor me by sitting in this audience tonight responded to an invitation for the fifteenth day of *November*, and I am sure you did not give a thought to how illogical it was on our part to invite you for the fifteenth day of the "ninth" month (mind you, "November" means ninth in Latin!) when November is actually the eleventh month.

Of course, this example of seemingly flagrant illogic has its justification in consensus: everybody calls this wintry month November. But it also has good historical reasons, and only these make the choice of the name for the month understandable. *September*, the month of the fall equinox, was, in fact, the seventh month (as the name indicates) as long as the new year started with *March*, the month of the vernal equinox, the month the sun enters Aries, the first of the twelve constellations of the zodiac. In the Hebrew calendar, the string of months still starts with Nissan (roughly March) making Tishri (roughly September) the seventh month. This type of reckoning was changed a few decades before the start of our common era when, to correct or replace the by that time utterly confused Roman calendar, Julius Caesar, a dictator of genius if there ever was one, decreed that the year start with the Calends of January, the month dedicated to the god Janus. And so it remained. In our present system of days and months, July and August (the names honor Caesar of the *gens Julia* and *Augustus*, the emperor who further improved on the solar calendar) are respectively the seventh and eighth months.

Caesar was a clever dictator; he never made any more changes than necessary. (He never called himself "emperor.") Thus, the month of the fall equinox retained its customary name: *September.* It seems that the system works quite well; in spite of the improper naming, you all, thank Heaven, gathered tonight. By common agreement, today *is* the fifteenth day of November. . . .

The second remark pertains to the title of my lecture, retained as the title of this essay. I confess, the word "dyslexia" was, in a way, chosen as an eye-catcher, as a term much *en vogue* nowadays. Availing myself of it was, in fact, justified only because I meant it in the broadest possible sense of the word, that is, as trouble or difficulty in reading or learning to read, without any qualifying adjectives. I must make it clear from the beginning that I do not plan to discuss so-called "true" ("primary" or "essential") dyslexia, possibly a hereditary disorder, the condition to which the term is restricted by some authorities. Nor will I discuss "symptomatic" reading disability, "neurological" reading disability caused by actual and very early brain damage, a condition to which authorities like Quadfasel and Goodglass (1968) attach the name "dyslexia" with hesitation. I have not seen enough of these cases. I have little firsthand information about either of these conditions. However, I am not alone in using the term "dyslexia" in such a broad sense. In a paper entitled "Dyslexia — a problem in definition," S. L. Rosner (1968) stated: "dyslexia, if indeed the term has any relevance, is a category which is first and foremost educational." Contributions of the neurologist, the psychologist, the psychiatrist, the vision specialist are, according to Rosner, "peripheral rather than central." He goes on to say that nothing much is gained by the statement that a child cannot learn to read because he is "dyslexic" when actually the diagnosis that he is "dyslexic" is based on the circumstance that he has trouble learning to read. This author continues: "When it comes right down to it, the youngster must receive treatment for dyslexia with a skilled remedial teacher."

In a word, I do mean any kind of inability to read or unsatisfactory reading ability when I speak of "dyslexia." For the purposes of this essay, "dyslexia" is a problem in learning, a problem to be overcome by teaching — nothing more.

Having a reputation as an expert on vision, I see quite a few poor readers, probably more than many of my colleagues. It is certainly not an illogical step on the part of parents and teachers to consult an ophthalmologist. Reading is, after all, an activity involving the eyes, and parents and teachers hope (often against hope) that what is wrong with the child who is a poor reader is the eyes. Sometimes something *is* wrong with the eyes, though generally not with eyesight. Children who have a visual problem due to some ocular pathology are clearly in the domain of the ophthalmologist. They need treatment if the condition is treatable. They need careful refraction, proper illumination, proper optical aids, books of large print, etc., to help them have better use of their remaining vision, once the loss is stationary. Many times, to my great satisfaction, I have been able to offer considerable help. Once in a while one or another of these children has become a retarded reader because of a purely visual handicap. But more often than not, children with poor eyesight are surprisingly good readers and one is often amazed how much they can accomplish with so little.

I have seen many children with high refraction error, astigmatism, even nystagmus,[2] who read well. I have also seen children with amblyopia in one eye who have no reading problem. Finally, I have seen many a poor reader with no or only minimal refraction error and 20/20 vision in both eyes. The children in the last category whom I as an eye specialist have really been able to help generally had trouble with binocular coordination. One does not have to have good vision, specifically good distance vision, in order to be a good reader. Myopes are notoriously good readers. One does not have to use both eyes in order to be a good reader. But one must be free of eyestrain, a clearcut entity, however nebulous the term. A cross-eyed child never suffers from eyestrain, not, at least, on account of the strabismus. A cross-eyed child may be a poor reader, but not because he is cross-eyed. Let me just mention two cases, two extremes, that I have seen lately.

A 7-year-old boy with nystagmus, no apparent retinal pathology and no significant refraction error was sent to me by a Long Island ophthalmologist on account of learning difficulties. The boy turned out to be a binocular amblyope, his amblyopia being a symptom regularly associated with so-called typical total color blindness. His handicap made it impossible for him to adjust to a regular well-lit, often overbright, school environment. (This type of child just cannot function under daylight conditions or bright illumination. Bright light blinds him.) He had failed to learn to read. Reasoned suggestions to parents and school authorities greatly remedied the situation.

Such a case is, of course, a rare exception and not really a case of dyslexia of either variety, though the boy's nystagmus suggested brain damage to the school psychologist.

A high-school student (let me add, a brilliant young man) while in elementary school suffered such agonies when doing any close work that for years he stayed behind his age group in learning to read. He was really a retarded reader, but had been classified as mentally retarded. This boy had high myopia and esophoria with poor ability to keep his eyes straight. He had eyestrain. He maintained binocular vision with great difficulty. Still he could not help maintaining it. The compulsion to "fusion" (to using the two eyes together) was too great. I made this young man happy for a while with prisms but ultimately operated on his overacting medial rectus muscles.

This was an example of so-called dyslexia that an ophthalmologist and only an ophthalmologist could cure.

If I mention a third case, it is largely because of the peculiar setting.

A 10-year-old boy came to see me with his worried and not very young parents recently. As it turned out, the father was (of all things) chairman of the department of psychology in one of our prestigious midwestern universities. The boy ate with the left hand and threw a ball with the left hand, but wrote with the right hand. He was a somewhat retarded reader and subject (or subjected) to all possible help the vision experts in the department could muster, from visual perceptual training (there was nothing wrong with visual perception) and stereoscopic exercises (he has good stereopsis) to convergence drills (he overconverged). It turned out that this poor overtreated boy had esophoria (tendency to converge the eyes) for distance, convergence excess (greater esophoria for near than for distance), and moderate hypermetropia (what is called farsightedness). (This is the most common triad of ocular functional abnormalities in poor readers.) The boy also had fatigue diplopia, a symptom which seemed most alarming to everyone. (It is one of the "soft" neurologic signs.) Visual acuity was normal in both eyes. Bifocals, to be worn constantly, were prescribed. This eliminated the convergence excess and prevented diplopia. I am quite sure it has helped his reading.

I have had several patients with reading difficulties in which aniseikonia, the inequality of the images in the two eyes, made it hard for the two eyes to cooperate. These were cases of eyestrain which a proper optical correction helped to relieve. Eyestrain from whatever cause in those crucial years in which a child has to learn to read often leads to a distaste for reading, and if these years are not fully utilized it becomes hard to catch up later. Frustration, resentment, teachers' disapproval, parents' apprehension, schoolmates' ridicule, all add up to a psychological superstructure under which the real cause — the eyestrain — almost disappears. These are the cases Quadfasel and Goodglass properly list under the heading "Secondary Reading Retardation." These cases probably constitute the majority of our patients with reading problems. And since they also form the group for which a lot can be done, they are the cases that deserve our utmost effort. By all means, children with reading problems should be seen by an ophthalmologist, and if there is a refraction error of sufficient magnitude, it should be corrected. Especially careful attention should be paid to ocular muscular imbalance, the main cause of eyestrain and a frequent cause of secondary reading retardation. If it is found that aniseikonia may be a factor, this should be corrected.

I am a great believer in correction of ocular muscular imbalance with prisms (also in some cases with bifocals), and as I mentioned I am less hesitant than most of my colleagues to operate on patients with muscular imbalance of small degree if symptoms justify it. Often coordination has its peculiarities. If a child is patently cross-eyed, if one can see the strabismus from the other side of the street, he can be sure that this child has no eyestrain. This child has solved his problems by breaking up binocular coordination. He uses one eye exclusively or one eye at a time. But if imbalance is of merely 3 or 5 degrees, as in the cases I have just mentioned, then the child makes a constant, compulsive subconscious effort during all of his waking hours to keep eyes straight and binocular vision operative in spite of the eyes' tendency to turn. Here optical correction or — if it does not solve the problem — surgery, minimal surgery, is in order.

Having had the opportunity to see so many children with reading difficulties, I want to mention one point, and that is that an inordinate number are lefthanded among them. I shall return to this point later. Having been a practicing physician with a sympathetic ear I have also become familiar with the dilemmas of modern, mid-twentieth-century, upper-middle-class parents whose attitude toward their children is a lamentable mixture of permissiveness, uncertainty, and guilt feeling. Nothing exonerates these poor guilt-ridden parents as much as the diagnosis of so-called specific dyslexia or minimum brain damage, hidden birth injury, and strephosymbolia, and, of course, perceptual immaturity (the correction of which by exercises with impressive machinery has become one of the blooming businesses of paramedicine). What can these poor parents do if the child's brain has failed to develop proper lateral dominance, proper directional orientation, proper *Gestalt* recognition, etc.?! They are so happy to spend money on people who can cure all this by oscillating orthoptic equipment or by letting their little patients crawl on the floor. However, the more cases of retarded reading ability I see, the more I am convinced that one of the main sources of trouble is poor teaching methods.

Perhaps I exaggerate. But with Dr. Rudolf Flesch, author of the famous (many call it notorious) book *Why Johnny Can't Read* (1955), and a fortunately growing number of educators, I feel that what has produced the appalling number of poor readers in American schools in the last decades (many more than "primary" dyslexia or neurologic reading retardation should account for) is the "look-and-say" method of teaching reading. Yes, "look-and-see-the-meaning" *is* the ultimate goal of the efficient reader. It is the ultimate reward that, after difficult beginnings, English spelling can bestow upon the one who reads. But at first a child has to learn how to write and pronounce English sound symbols (the technical term is "graphemes") and what the rules are for spelling English words.

As I mentioned earlier in this introduction, communication is based on consensus. But this consensus is understandable only in terms of history. Writing and reading as well as speaking and listening are our main means of communication. The meaning of the sounded word and the sound value of the written word are both based on agreements, and these agreements all have a history. Only through an analysis of their history can the rules or peculiarities (whatever you call them) of English spelling offer themselves to comprehension — unless we believe that English spelling is nothing but a whimsical brainchild of Doctor Johnson (who, if such was the case, should never have been born).

I have in the past years slowly come to the conclusion that my job as a vision expert has been mostly didactic. I seldom have the opportunity to teach teachers how to teach, but most parents are cooperative and willing to take a hand. Thus over the past ten or fifteen years I have developed a system of spelling comprehension which I have tried to share with parent and child, and which I shall try to present in the chapters that follow. This system actually grew on me, unplanned, as more and more children with reading problems flocked into my office. I never meant to develop one. I have, of course, also been interested — for many years — in the history of writing and of languages, and another purpose of this essay besides the one I have just mentioned is sharing some of the pleasure, excitement, and enlightenment my studies have given me over the years.

NOTES

[1]These introductory remarks are taken, practically verbatim, from my Semmelweis-award lecture (given November 15, 1968), which explains the form in which they are presented.

[2]A glossary of terms which a nonophthalmologist might possibly have difficulty in understanding appears at the end of the book.

CHAPTER ONE

The Different Meanings of the Word H-A-T — The History of the Letters H and T — The Biology of Righthandedness — The Silent E — Phonograms vs. Ideograms — "Code" vs. "Meaning"

Let me begin with a simple example, a word consisting of three "phonemes" if we look at it as a spoken utterance, or of three "graphemes" (three sound symbols, three letters) if our attention is turned toward the written word. A phoneme is an element of human speech. Phonemes can only be heard, not looked upon. That I used the phrase "if we look at it" is, obviously, just a convenient figure of speech. What one can show in print or on a blackboard are not phonemes but graphemes, symbols of phonemes, sound symbols, letters, in this instance three letters:

H-A-T

We agree that each of these marks is the symbol of a certain sound, and we also agree that in pronouncing them we are going to start from the left.

Language, writing, reading, are matters of agreement, first of all. I cannot repeat this often enough. Spoken language can serve communication only if there is agreement on the meaning of the spoken words which are sequences of uttered sounds. Written language can serve communication only if there is agreement on both the sound value of each of the written symbols and on the direction of our scanning across them.

There is, of course, reason behind these latter agreements.

Every one of our written symbols has a history. It was not just someone's whim that the first symbol on the left became a command to
utter the sound of breathing, the sound /h/.[1] In its long history the
symbol was first an ideogram. It symbolized a *fence* (KHETH in
Hebrew[2]), two vertical posts with one or two or more bars across. In
the course of its further development, the symbol of the fence became the symbol of the sound that starts the Semitic word for fence,
the symbol for the sound /kh/. The Greeks made a vowel symbol
(H) out of it (they retained the form but changed the essence), a symbol for a vowel sound pronounced like a long English /ā/ in HATE.
(They called it ÉTA.) Finally, through Latin writing, it became a symbol for the sound of breathing. Linguists call it an aspirate. Whatever,
however, the history of the letter, we now pronounce it like /h/ in the
German HABEN, and that is what we teach our children. We tell
them that this pattern *is* pronounced as /h/. The third symbol, again
by agreement, tells us to press our tongue to the back of our teeth
while exhaling. Linguists speak of an "alveolar stop" or, to be more
accurate, a "voiceless alveolar stop." Again there is a history to the
letter. TAV in Hebrew is the word for *cross*, and the form of the letter
(t or T) stuck to the form of the ideogram almost unchanged over
three millennia. But this again does not matter. We have agreed to
sound the voiceless alveolar stop /t/ when we see this sound symbol,
and our children just have to accept this. In teaching it is the teacher
and not the student who calls the tune. No majority of rebellious
undergraduates will, I hope, prevail in forcing us to sound this sign
as, say, an /r/. This would lead to a breakdown of communication. It
would be the beginning of the end of civilization. Reading, like speaking, is a matter of conventions. We must agree that a certain symbol
represents a certain sound and that the directed conglomeration of
certain sounds means a certain thing or act, or quality — whichever
it may be. The word "directed" is important. It involves a time element. The three phonemes

$$\longrightarrow \quad /d/\text{-}/o/\text{-}/g/ \quad \longleftarrow$$

when pronounced in the direction indicated by the arrow on the left
symbolize one thing; pronounced in the direction symbolized by the
other arrow, they mean something entirely different. Agreement and
acceptance come first; understanding can only follow.

About the history of the middle letter I shall not say anything at present. We all agree that it is a sound symbol for a vowel. We also all agree, as I have already stated, that in pronouncing the three sound symbols we shall start with the one on the left. Composing written words from written letters we transform time into space. Left for the English reader means "Begin!" But this too is purely a matter of agreement. The symbols could just as well be "read" from right to left. Reading them in this manner might, however, convey no meaning or some other meaning. The three sound symbols H-A-T could convey no meaning were they read from right to left; the three sound symbols D-O-G would have a different meaning from the one intended. We have to agree on a direction, and our children have to be taught the direction. Reading is not looking. Whatever modern educators say, we do not "*look*-and-say," we *scan*-and-say. Reading is scanning. It is an activity with a direction, just as speaking is.

Again, there are good historical reasons, even good biological reasons, to support the choice of direction that our ancestors came to make for us. Ever since the dawn of our race's history, the right hand has been the hand of aggression, and the left hand the hand of protection. The shield was worn by the left hand to protect the heart, which is on the left side. The spear was worn by the right hand, the easier to attack the opponent's heart, which is straight in line with the spear. In the struggle for existence those holding the spear in the right hand have prevailed. They are in the clear majority. And since the right hand is the hand of aggression, all tools are now geared for the right hand; screws turn toward the right; the cutting blade of scissors works through the right thumb; the handle of the scythe is swung by the right arm; the brush of the painter and the bow of the violinist are held in the right hand. The stylus with which our Sumerian, Persian, Minoan ancestors made their cuneiform marks was also held by the right hand. So now the right hand is also the hand of skills, of manipulation and articulation. When the right hand became the hand of skills, the left brain had to become the matrix behind the skills.[3] Some eight percent of people are lefthanded, but when it comes to language, to speech, even lefthanded people are more often leftbrained than rightbrained (Goodglass and Quadfasel, 1954). Writing with the right hand is, thus, biologically determined. *We write with the right hand because our heart is on the left side.* It is the outcome of natural selection. Starting to write on the left side of the page is, on the other hand, purely a convention, a matter of convenience.

Using wet clay as the material to write on, the righthanded scribe must have soon found out that the best way to avoid smudging over what he had just written was by starting at the upper left corner of the tablet. Cuneiforms, therefore, mostly start at the upper left. So do some Egyptian hieroglyphics. But this is not a *sine qua non* for giving meaning to writing. On the contrary, with all its mechanical advantages, writing from left to right with the right hand is a secondary arrangement. The columns in Chinese script follow from right to left.[4] My Semitic ancestors also retained the original, though technically much poorer, choice. Hebrew and Arabic are still written from right to left, though with the right hand. Israelites, of course, were never much given to experimentation.[5] That was the forte of the Greeks. It was the Greeks who, after first writing from right to left, then writing in both directions (they even had a beautiful name, *Boustrophedon*, for it), finally decided on the direction left to right. Be this as it may, writing and reading could just as well be a scanning procedure, a vectorial affair, directed from right to left. In the end, it is purely a matter of agreement that English is written from left to right, a matter for the teacher to teach and to enforce. The accepted and agreed way in our Western civilization is to write and to read from left to right — and to write with the right hand. As I shall try to explain later, we are doing our lefthanded children a questionable favor by letting them write with the left hand. I know many lefthanded people, but I have never yet seen a lefthander who played the fiddle with the left hand.[6] Has one of my psychoanalyst friends ever had the chance to analyze a lefthanded cellist or violinist? Has this man's ego suffered? We ought to know. There are (this at least is the way I feel about it) too many people around us who write with the left hand. Is it possible that some of them symbolize parental insecurity and permissiveness, a breakdown of authority, and an unfortunate educational psychology rather than an increasing prevalance of true lefthandedness?

Let me return to the three characters H-A-T and present my main argument against the look-and-say method. It will not be difficult to convince anyone that these three symbols, while they symbolize three phonemes in proper order, in no way symbolize, in themselves, any kind of object or action. They have no "meaning." But this is what our children have been taught for the last quarter of a century, and this is, of course, why so many of them don't know how to read. They are taught to look and not to scan. They are taught to associate meaning, not with the ordered arrangement of sounds which these letters symbolize, but with the visual image of the printed word. Moreover, what is most lamentable, they are taught to read first, not to write first. They don't see that written words, like spoken words, run in time and don't stand still in space.[7]

In reality, the three patterns we are still discussing here symbolize three sounds in a given order and this is all. It is the three sounds in a given order that symbolize a thing or action. And this is of tremendous importance. There is no short-cut to meaning, whatever educational psychologists might tell us to the contrary. It is the spoken word that is the symbol of a thing or act. A child must learn that these three written symbols are to be pronounced ⟶ /h/-/a/-/t, in this sequence, and only if the child speaks English will the pronounced word mean an object to cover one's head with. It is not the three written characters that symbolize that object.

It so happens that the simple sequence of three phonemes (a meaningful sequence of phonemes is called, by linguists, a morpheme) means different things in a number of languages. In English, of course, it means the object one uses to cover one's head with. In German (the vowel is pronounced with a slight variation) the morpheme signifies something entirely different:

ER HAT = HE HAS

and signifies possession. It is the third person singular of the auxiliary verb HABEN. In Swedish, my friends tell me, the word means what in English would be HATE and in German would be HASS. The three words are "cognate"; they have the same origin.

Approximately the same morpheme listened to by a Frenchman will for the latter symbolize what the English would call HASTE and what in German is HAST. Of course, the French will spell the word somewhat differently:

HÂTE

and will also pronounce it with a fine difference. Still, the fact that the Frenchman says that he is

À LA HÂTE

and not

À L'HÂTE

when he is "in a hurry," indicates that the H is a phoneme to be pronounced while the little tent on top of the A is just a reminder that once upon a time there was another consonant in the word, an S, that is still present in both the English cognate HASTE and the German cognate HAST. Frenchmen, like Englishmen, are historically minded people and their spelling peculiarities are always (well, almost always) explicable in historical terms. A few pertinent examples are:

CHÂTEAU	CASTLE	CASTRUM
HÔTEL	HOSTEL	
ARRÊT	ARREST	
FENÊTRE		FENESTRA
ÎSLE	ISLAND	INSULA
MAÎTRE	MASTER	MAGISTER
NÔTRE		NOSTER
SÛR	SURE	SECURUS

Crowded consonants add a quality of harshness to the language which the French, for instance, try to avoid.

The same three letters signal three homophones in Hungarian only one of which is of any interest to us, HAT, which means 6 in Hungarian.

The fact that

$$HAT = SIX = 6$$

gives me the opportunity to remind the readers that there indeed exists an entirely different class of written symbols, symbols that are independent of the spoken word. These symbols we call *ideograms* as opposed to the *phonograms* that make up most of ordinary written language. Ideograms are what the Chinese use. Ideograms, of course, were the beginning of all writing. It took centuries, possibly millennia, for a syllabic and then a phonemic writing to develop out of ideograms; it took time for the symbol of an ox (ALEPH in Hebrew means ox) finally to become the graphem still called *aleph* in Hebrew, still called *alpha* in Greek, and now called A, the middle letter in our H-A-T.

We have retained some ideographs in our writing. More accurately, we have fabricated some. We use $ for DOLLAR, lb for POUND, Na for SODIUM. Letter groups like IBM, LSD, DNA are by now understood in all languages, and the swastika or the hammer and sickle (Fig. 1) have the same connotation to all of us, whatever the language we are thinking in. But only in our notation of numbers have we retained a true semblance, if only a semblance, of that Eden-like condition in which every man understood every other man's tongue. Written symbols like

$$6 + 4 = 10 \qquad \text{or} \qquad 10 = 4 + 6$$

can be read in any language and in both directions, and until our children came home with their embarrassing "new mathematics" textbooks, we parents believed that these symbols can have only one meaning. What in Hungarian is called HAT is SIX for the French and the Englishman, SECHS for a German, SHISHA for the Hebrew, but all will understand the written numerals. Written numerals are independent of the sound groups that each language secondarily hangs upon these concepts. Of course, these

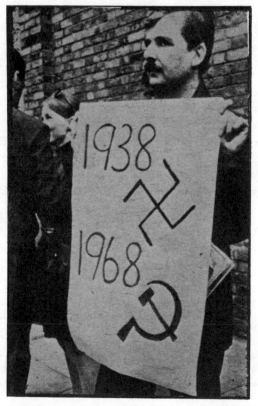

Fig. 1. Ideograms. Numbers and symbols that mean the same in any language.

concept symbols, the numerals, can also serve their purpose only if there is agreement as to their meaning. Numerals, too, grew to what they are today. They have a history and so has counting. Our numerals, from 2 to 9, are in my estimation modified Semitic letter symbols,[8] and *ten* is the basis of our generally accepted "decimal" system of calculation, the algorithm, because we happen to have ten fingers. The written symbol 10 (one and zero) means *ten* only as long as we *give* it this meaning. As our children are now taught in their new mathematics, the written symbol 10 (one and zero) can equally well mean *eight* or *twelve* if we are to calculate in an octal or a duodecimal system (or, in fact, any other number) and means *two* in the most revolutionary of all newer systems, the binary system, upon which computer technology is built. Nor is there a problem of "true" or "false" involved. The notation

$$5 + 5 = 10 \qquad 5 + 5 + 5 + 5 = 20$$

may appear to us so familiar as to be self-evident. Still the notations

(Octal)	$4 + 4 = 10$	$4 + 4 + 4 + 4 = 20$
(Duodecimal)	$6 + 6 - 10$	$6 + 6 + 6 + 6 - 20$
(Binary)	$1 + 1 = 10$	$1 + 1 + 1 + 1 = 100$

are no less "true," each of them in its peculiar system of reckoning. *Agreement* is the basis of each and every form of communication, including calculation, but only through its *history* can we understand why any symbol, be it number or letter or ideogram, came to mean what it does. Nor does history prove that we have always made the best choice. Making *ten* the basis of our algorithm has its good biological reason, the fact that we have ten fingers. (Twenty, the number of fingers and toes combined, survives in "score" and in "quatre-vingt.") But as all students of numberology (forgive the term) know, a duodecimal system of counting, if generally accepted, would have been far superior. It speaks for the rationality of Anglo-Saxon thinking that the British have until recently been so tenacious in not submitting to the decimal system, and in keeping to a basis of twelves — the dozen, the foot of twelve inches, the troy pound of twelve ounces, the shilling of twelve pence. Indeed, counting in twelves stayed with us through the ages in spite of our fingers. We find it natural that the clockface carries twelve numbers. Astrologers read twelve constellations. Even the most radical calendar reformer would hold on to the twelve-month year. Much of biblical lore revolved around the number twelve. Israel had twelve sons, the Savior had twelve apostles, Christmas has twelve days. Only of the Commandments (most of them don'ts) were there ten.

But let me return to the French variant of my three phonemes which, in writing, took four letters:

HÂTE

In the written form we have a letter, the letter E, that is not the equivalent, the counterpart of a phoneme. It is not a sound sign; it is a command signal. It tells the reader that the letter *to the left* of this signal (mark, please, the essential feature: to the *left* of this signal) must be pronounced. Were this signal missing, the pronunciation would change. Thus, while the little tent over the A primarily has historical justification and does not essentially affect pronunciation, the E has a job to fulfill. It is not really a letter. The French Academy could, if it saw reason for it, decide that in the future this so-called "silent E" is to be replaced by, say, an asterisk, HAT*. To repeat: the letter E in HÂTE is not really a letter, not a sound sign. It is not a symbol but a signal, a modifier. In the temporal sequence of ocular scanning, what the modifier modifies is in front of the modifier, not behind it.

Now let us see the same arrangement of letters without the tent, the *accent circonflexe*. This gives us an English word of four written letters:

H-A-T-E

while the morpheme which these four letters signify again consists of only three phonemes. We once more meet that so-called "silent E," which in this case modifies the sound value of a letter placed two steps to the left. The scanning gaze of the English eye has to stop in what should be its even and uniform flow from left to right over the written or printed line; it has to rebound to a sound signal *two* steps to the left, to a component the pronunciation of which hangs fire until the modifier has caught the eye and has said its say. A Hungarian or a Czech child, in the blessed simplicity of the spelling of his language, would not for a moment hesitate to pronounce the word as two syllables,

HA-TE

the second following the first in normal sequence. The English child is expected to do much more. No sooner has the English child been taught to utter the sound /a/ when he sees the letter A — what we might call the "basic" sound value of the letter A — in words like

HAT   FAT   MAT   RAT   etc.

than he is asked to do differently. He is, in fact, asked to suspend the execution of an action he has just been taught to perform until more information has become available, until more of the circumstances have crystallized.

I cannot help wanting to use the adjective "formidable" in connection with such a requirement. It is a truly formidable task for both teacher and child. *It is not easy to learn to read English. It is not easy to teach reading in English.* But let me add that there is hardly anything that, to a latecomer to the English language, as I am, better explains one of the most sublime qualities of Anglo-Saxon civilization. While learning to read English, a child learns to suspend action,[9] even to suspend judgment, until added information is available, until more of the circumstances have crystallized.

In learning to read, no such problem faces the Hungarian child. In addition to the word HAT that I analyzed earlier, Hungarian also has a word HÉT, meaning WEEK or SEVEN, which sounds just like the English HATE we are now discussing. Hungarian orthography manages without the help of a silent E by having created a vowel symbol sign É for /ā/.[10] Hungarian also has a word HÁT (meaning BACK in English). In this word the vowel sounds like /āh/, somewhat like the one in English BAR. English spelling has no immediately apparent way to indicate that the vowels in HAT, HATE, BAR, BARE, and SAW are not identical. Having not found any use for diacritical signs, it had to resort to retroacting modifiers for the purpose. Hungarian or Czech writing does not apply such devices and does not face the problems that make English spelling so difficult but in the long run so full of sense. English spelling imbues the written word with meaning. Its peculiarities, its seeming irregularities, transform English phonograms into quasi-ideograms without at the same time destroying the essentially sequential character of their elements.

It seems as if with such a statement we acknowledge the at least partial correctness of the look-and-say method, of what, in a more conciliatory vein, we might call the "meaning" method of teaching reading as opposed to the "code" method (Chall, 1967). This is indeed the case. Things never are pure black or pure white. Certainly a technique of teaching reading that, after all, has prevailed for decades cannot be entirely wrong. It must have proved to be at least partially successful, and the philosophy behind it must contain certain elements of truth. Admittedly, most pupils do learn to read well and efficiently when subjected to this technique (or philosophy) of teaching. Besides, the two techniques must have many features in common since both aim at the same goal. They cannot be mutually exclusive.

On the one hand, written or printed English words are — as I have just intimated — more than pure phonograms in great many instances, and the sooner we make our pupils aware of this fact, the more purposeful and the more successful will be our teaching. On the other hand, even the most ardent followers of the see-meaning-at-a-glance technique teach, must teach, some phonics. But even if they do not — which is unthinkable — they will not, and cannot, prevent their pupils from picking up the elements of phonics by whatever incidental means. A child will learn (even if he is not taught it) that in the sight complex[11] HAT, whatever its meaning, there is a picture element H that means just the sound /h/ and nothing else, and a picture element T that means just the sound /t/ and nothing else. Furthermore, the child cannot fail to note, unless he is mentally retarded, that in the sight forms HAT, HIT, HOT, HUT, and HATE, whatever their meaning, certain elements are common and others not. Moreover, even if sight reading is the order of the day, the child will, and must, find out that the sighting of the H element occurs somehow, for some reason, *before* the sighting of the T element — whether in time or space the child will not bother to analyze. Finally, the child cannot fail to note that in the "ideograms" TOP and POT the picture elements, taken one by one, are all identical, each representing one particular sound, that what is not identical is just their order, and that the "proper" order is not a matter of seeing but of agreement or (in case of the teaching/learning situation) of instruction. Word pictures are pictures, but pictures with direction (a time element) built in, because they consist of phonic symbols. No teacher of English can question the fact that English written or printed words consist of elements that, *one by one*, are phonic symbols. Thus, everybody does teach phonics.

Even if all this (the elements of phonics) were not taught and words were presented as timeless *Gestalten* (much as Chinese writing is generally presented to the Western reader[12]), the idea of order, of regulated sequence in space and time, must still be communicated. Individual, meaningful, written or printed word *Gestalten* can be strung into meaningful statements only if (1) these words are ordered into some agreed-upon sequence (in the case of English in horizontal rows from left to right, in the case of Chinese from top downward), and if (2) these rows of words are stacked in an agreed-upon sequence (in the case of English from top to bottom, in the case of Chinese

from right to left). However little we think of it, all these are significant elements of agreement in instruction — whatever the philosophy
of the teacher and his or her teaching technique. English printed sentences, whether one "sight" — reads the component words or not,
are to be read from left to right in rows that follow from above down-
wards. As far as writing is concerned, even the most ardent adherent
to the "meaning" approach will consider it absurd to let a child write
individual words, such as the "ideogram" AMERICAN, starting
from the right. (For a true *Gestalt* reader, who allegedly looks at word
pictures for meaning and is oblivious to sound and direction, this
should not really matter.) Writing *is* an activity in space as well as in
time. Words are written from left to right, and the word

→ *American*

is *written* in a sequence that just cannot be changed and which even a
lefthander must follow.

Vice versa, we must concede that a great many English words
(especially the so-frequent monosyllabic homophones) can only be
handled efficiently if in addition to the sound of the word its written
or printed word picture is also considered. We can do this readily. It
will not change the fact that reading, and especially spelling, English
words can be taught much better by a phonics technique, by making
the pupil look for a "code," for the *keys to pronunciation* in the
ordered sequence of the written or printed word elements. There are
generally more letters than phonemes to an English word. There are
four graphic elements in the written word

HATE

but only three sounds in the morpheme they represent. The extra
letter is the pronunciation signal, the retroactive modifier, a visual
element. One should not perplex the mind of an inquisitive child by
telling him that the E is "silent" and no more. A silent letter makes no
sense to the unbending logic of a child. He should be told what the
extra letter is doing, not what it is not doing, even if out of habit we
call it "silent."

With all of this double-coding system, the sound elements and
the modifiers, English words still need to be sounded out. They have
to be "scanned over," not "looked at." A space sequence has to be
translated into a time sequence. In this respect English written words

are like all other written words in all other alphabetically written languages. English written words, too, are, first of all, symbols of morphemes. Only *secondarily*, through experience, do English written words also acquire the quality of quasi-ideograms.

This added "seen meaning" of English written words can be best demonstrated in the example of so-called homophones to which I have already referred. In the example

NITE   KNIGHT   (/n/-/ī/-/t/)

(for which I apologize — I despise "reformed" spelling) we are provided with a purely visual factor (the letters-in-sequence) which conveys to us the intended meaning of the morpheme. (The latter, the sounded word, is, of course, the *same* in both instances.)

The eventually emerging pattern of quasi-ideograms in which the English language abounds has in reality little to do with the *pseudo-*ideograms of the look-and-say technique. Look-and-see-the-meaning-of-a-word is not the short-cut modern reading teachers had hoped for. It is the experienced reader's ultimate reward.

NOTES

[1] Lower-case letters between diagonals / / are used to represent phonemes, individual sound elements of speech.

[2] I am not a linguist or philologist and must be forgiven by experts if in the course of this discussion I use the term "Hebrew" much too often and somewhat indiscriminately. Hebrew and (to an even less degree) Aramaic are the only Semitic tongues somewhat familiar to me, and inadvertently I use the word "Hebrew" as almost equivalent with "Semitic." I am aware that the major part of the credit for the invention of alphabetic writing goes to the Phoenicians, another Semitic tribe. As far as this discussion is concerned, my inaccuracy will not matter.

Much of my knowledge of the history of these symbols comes from the book *The 26 Letters* by Oscar Ogg (New York, Crowell, 1948), who correctly refers to Phoenician and Egyptian sources in his history of the 26 letters of the English alphabet.

[3] Why the image of the right half of the world is projected upon the left brain, why the left brain governs the right hand, and why, ultimately, speech, the most articulate of human skills, is also governed by the left brain, are attractive problems which I cannot now discuss. (See my book, *Physiology of the Eye*, Volume II, *Vision*, New York, Grune & Stratton, 1952, for some comments. Also see Appendixes A and B of this book.)

Why the heart, man's heart, is asymmetrically located, and on the left side, is, of course, the problem of problems. However, to ponder over it would lead me even farther astray. (Those interested in such questions will find much pleasure in M. Gardner's delightful *The Ambidextrous Universe*, Pelican, 1970.)

[4]A few remarks on Chinese writing are to be found later in this book.

[5]To explain why Hebrew writing starts from the right, one could also mention that the Lord carved the Ten Commandments onto stone tablets, not tablets of clay. He must have done it with hammer and chisel, and he must have held the hammer in the right hand. There was no problem of smudging: there was no reason for him not to start on the more natural side, the right side. (One must, of course, assume that the Lord is righthanded. It took a woman, Mme Simone de Beauvoir, to assume that God is a "She." But no one has so far suggested that He or She is lefthanded.) By the way, the language the Lord used was Hebrew, we assume, and this is the reason why some of the Founding Fathers seriously thought of making Hebrew the official language of these United States. There are, though, some doubts possible. An early nineteenth century monk and professor of history at the University of Pesth, one István Horvát, wrote a treatise in which from an analysis of biblical proper names he deduced that the Lord's own language was — you guessed it — Hungarian.

[6]A seeming (but only seeming) exception to this statement will be discussed in Chapter Nine.

[7]For this, of course, we cannot solely blame the "method." Our children are nowadays surrounded by print. Neon signs, signs in shop windows, inscriptions on packagings and containers, newspapers, books, magazines, television are part and parcel of the urbanized ambiance which constantly hammers upon children's eyes. While speaking still comes as the challenge and listening as the answer in the natural order of events, reading has now all but evicted writing from its historic prime position. But this makes it even more imperative that we teach our children the vectorial character of the written letter and the written word. (More will be said about this later.)

[8]To me the similarity between the so-called Arabic numerals 2 to 9 and the Hebrew letters of the same numerical value is so obvious that I am reluctant to carry coals to Newcastle and therefore relegate this information to a footnote. I am sure others must have pointed out this similarity long ago. The books on the history of the alphabet I have had a chance to read did not. All, of course, mention the fact that the ancient Hebrews and Greek had no algorithm and no separate numerals, and that they used letters in alphabetic order conveniently to indicate our numbers 1, 2, 3, . . ., 10, 20, 30, . . ., 100, 200, etc., and combinations of them for other numbers. (כ, the eleventh letter, stands for "twenty" in Hebrew; ד, the fourth letter, stands for "four"; thus, כד is "twenty-four.")

Our numeral "one" is an exception. While the letter ALEPH does symbolize the numeral "one" in Hebrew (in addition to signifying some lost consonant sound), our numeral for "one" is just a digit, a vertical line; it has no relation to ALEPH or ALPHA. But that the Hebrew letter for the sound /b/, the second letter of the Hebrew alphabet, is identical with our numeral for "two" — of that, I think, there can be no doubt. The Hebrew word BET means "house" — a floor, a wall, a roof, and a door. They are all there in the second letter of the Hebrew alphabet, the ideogram for a house: ב . Comparing it with our numeral 2 (Arabic ٢)

one will not doubt that the two patterns are the same. (The Arabic numeral is just turned 90 degrees.)

The third letter in the Hebrew alphabet is GIMEL, for "camel." The original symbol must have been η or Ν or ʍ — legs, a hump, a long neck. That the Hebrew ⅾ (script) or ⅾ (print) and the Latin G are cognate with

our numeral 3 or 3 (Arabic ٣)

is beyond question. The Hebrew letters run from right to left; the Latin letter is turned upside down; our numeral is the ideogram of the camel turned 90 degrees; the Arabic numeral is turned once more.

Similar is the relationship between the Hebrew alphabet's fourth letter, the name of which is DALET, for "door" — a vertical pivot and a horizontal bar.

Our numeral is 4 (the Arabic is ٤),

the cognate Hebrew letter is ٦ (script) or ٦ (print), while the Arabic numeral is the mirror image of the Hebrew ٦. A similar obvious relationship exists between

our numeral 6

and the Hebrew letter ٩, the name of which is VAV, for "club." Or between

our numeral 7 (Arabic V)

and the seventh Hebrew letter, ZAYYIN for "weapon." The Hebrew letters are ٢ (script), ٢ (print); the Greek and Latin ζ and Z, respectively, borrowed the form almost unchanged.

Our numeral 8 (Arabic Λ)

will be of special interest since we have already become acquainted with the eighth letter of the Hebrew alphabet, KHETH, the "fence." A fence, as I said, consists of at least two vertical bars, though the number and position of the horizontal bars is variable. The "fence" is still recognizable in the Hebrew ⴄ, the Greek η, and the Latin H. It had the form ♯ or ⊟ in the old Phoenician alphabet from which our number 8 directly derives. The corners got rounded off, and it can all be written with one stroke.

I would have to stretch imagination too far to find any relation between

our numeral 5

and the corresponding Hebrew letter HÉ = ⴄ. It looks more like the mirror image of the fifth Arabic letter, ⴄ, also called HÉ.

Our numeral 9 (Arabic ٩)

and the ninth Hebrew letter, THET, a "bundle of thread," also look quite unlike but only on first sight. In fact, our numeral is nothing but the Hebrew script letter THET = ⴜ turned upside down. And once the relationship is established, the printed Hebrew THET and the Greek THETA = θ appear obvious cognates with the numeral.

Here the parallelism ends. Our conventional written symbol for TEN is 10 or more accurately "10.", and this has nothing to do with the tenth Hebrew, Arabic, or Greek letter, or the X of the Latins. The algorithm and the ZERO were still unknown when Hebrews, Arabs, Greeks, and Romans developed their numbering systems.

The symbol for ZERO and the concept of "place" (the "decimal point") is, of course, one of the greatest mathematical inventions of all time. It is worth knowing that we immortalize their inventor, Al-Khvarizmi, with the term "algorithm."

[9]With all my boundless admiration for Anglo-Saxon civilization I once, in conversing on the subject, permitted myself the quip: "No wonder Anglo-Saxons suffer so much from constipation . . . "

[10]Actually it followed the French lead: É in French also sounds like /ā/.

[11]We might even use the term *Gestalt*.

[12]About this element in Chinese ideograms, see Chapter Eleven.

CHAPTER TWO

Intermezzo: A Dialogue with the Teacher — The "Irregular" Spelling of English Words — On Some Differences Between Vowels and Consonants — English Spelling: A Heroic Attempt to Meet Contradictory Challenges

The "silent E" is only one, the simplest one, of those retroactive determinants that are so characteristic of English spelling. Children have to be made familiar with the concept of the retroactive determinant at the earliest possible stage of the learning-to-read process. It enables them to solve hundreds of words on their own, and note, please, the word "*solve.*" A child has to learn to *solve* words, not to *recognize* individual words. When a boy of eight, looking at a word, tells me "I don't know that word" or "I have not yet learned this word," my heart contracts. That child has been done incalculable harm, and it makes no difference how many words he has learned to recognize in the first year. He has not been taught the technique of challenging words, of solving words! He has not been taught to read!

We have it from no less authority than Dr. Jeanne S. Chall, professor of education, Harvard University (1967), that an average child in the *first* grade knows about 4000 spoken words,[1] while that same child, trained by what she calls the "meaning" technique, has, by the end of the third grade, learned, or been exposed to, no more than 1500 printed words. They are mostly simple words, mostly "irregularly spelled" words,[2] mostly words restricted to some kind of idealized suburban (white) "family interest" vocabulary, mostly words whose meaning is fully clear to a child when he enters school. No more than 1500 words, constantly repeated! Is there any need for a more serious indictment of the technique?! Imagine a child who at the end of three years of schooling does not recognize, in writing or on the printed page, nearly two-thirds of the words which have been familiar to him through hearing them for at least two years! Obviously, by the end of the third school year this child has acquired many more new morphemes (sound sequences, spoken words with meaning) in addition to the 4000. But he has as yet no bridges *from* the written or printed equivalents of most of these morphemes *to* the morphemes and *to* their meaning, unless he has built them on his own, the teacher's philosophy notwithstanding. What manacling of the mind! Just think of all the words which an enriched environment with TV and radio offers to the average middle-class American child by the time he has finished third grade! Just think of the following not at all randomly selected, long, and, I quite realize, difficult words:

DEMOCRAT	SENATE	NOMINATION
REPUBLICAN	CONGRESS	ELECTION
	CONVENTION	INAUGURATION
MINORITY	PARLIAMENT	CAPITOL
MAJORITY	CANDIDATE	CEREMONY
	PRESIDENT	

How often have our eight- or nine-year-old children heard these words in a year that happens to be an election year? Realize that, restricted by the look-and-say recognition technique to the so-called "family" interest words, they have not acquired the means to recognize any of these words in print! They have actually been held back from recognizing them!

Admittedly, all the words just quoted are "long" words, words from the Greco-Roman superstructure of the English language, concept words (not just names of things), words that are meaningful only within the conceptual framework of a grown-up society, words that a child in a rural community hardly had the opportunity to hear fifty years ago. But even this does not matter. Opponents of the phonics technique sometimes argue that by the phonics approach a child might learn how to spell and pronounce words he does not yet understand. What of it? There is certainly no harm in this. The fact that a child cannot understand some words he is able to read (= de-code = sound out = turn into a sound sequence) by the phonics technique is much less deplorable than the fact that he cannot read[3] (= recognize

visually) at the end of the third grade two-thirds of the spoken words
he understood two years earlier. No one can understand every written
word he sees. We all read to learn. We expect to acquire new insight,
knowledge, concepts, ideas, through reading. For this purpose we
have to know how to attack new words, words not yet known. That is
what the teaching of reading is all about. A child acquires no knowledge just by learning to recognize printed words whose meaning he
already knows when he hears them. Reading is for learning. It is
everybody's bitter road toward knowledge. But at first we all have to
learn to read. The reading teacher's principal job is to teach the child
how to read, to hand down a "code," to show how to "de-code."

The amazing fact is (and to this I shall return again and again)
that there is nothing easier than to attack, by the phonics technique,
those words which the look-and-say technique so gingerly avoids. The
true challenge for the phonics attack are the short words, the basic,
simple, family interest words with so-called irregular spelling. The
rest of it is child's play. Words like

KNIGHT and WRONG (silent consonants)
HATE and BAR (retroactive modifiers, silent or not)
HEART and BREAST (same vowel digraph, different sound value)
VEIN and VAIN (same sound value, different digraphs)

are knotty problems for phonics attack. Words like

PRE-SID-ENT or RE-PUB-LIC-AN[4]

are not. It is the phonics analysis of the former words which will
mainly occupy us in following chapters.

As it turns out, in the last analysis the "meaning" teacher and
the "phonics" teacher both teach practically the same words, mostly
short words — the "meaning" teacher because they are basic words,
"family interest" words, words that because of their "irregular"
spelling have to be visually individually recognized through constant
repetition, and the phonics teacher for just the opposite reasons,
because they are the words through which the genius of English
script best reveals itself and the intimate, sensible, and history-
based relationship between spelled and sounded English words can
be best approached, analyzed, understood, and appreciated.

A dialogue with the teacher about the word "irregular," with its special connotations for our present context, is in order at this stage of our discussion. It is a much misused word, one the teacher had better avoid. Children are serious beings; they crave law and order and expect us grown-ups to present rules. The term "irregularly spelled" is one of those saving excuses held out in justification of the look-and-say teaching technique. Its proponents assert that words like KNIGHT and WRONG, HEART and BREAST, must be recognized purely *on sight* because their spelling is "inexplicable," "follows no rule," is "irregular." Nothing is more disappointing to a child than the admission of "irregularity," and nothing is gained by the notion.

A three-year-old child understands the difference between

(I) EAT   (I) ATE

perfectly well when he hears the words. (What he hears is, of course, /ee/-/t/ and /ā/-/t/.) A pupil in second grade trained by the phonics technique will also easily "phonemicize" them when he sees them even if, perchance, he has never seen them in print before. All this child will be expected to apply are two of the elementary rules of phonics (assuming that the teacher has given them to him earlier):

1. The digraph EA usually sounds /ee/ (a rule we shall discuss later).

2. The silent word-end E transforms the preceding A into /ā/ (a rule we have already met).

The student should certainly find nothing irregular in either the spoken or the written form of these words. In fact, the two word forms offer one of the simplest, most impressive, most logical and most natural-sounding ways to communicate, via the spoken word, both the common and the distinctive features of two related actions. (It is all a matter of approach.) Both words are of the same basic structure, a *long vowel plus T*, and both refer to the partaking of food, but with an added connotation: the signaling of "tense" — past versus present. What is gained by calling any part of this arrangement irregular? Teach your pupils something positive. If there is anything to be learned from some particular feature of spelling or grammar, don't fail to tell them. Rather than tell your students that such and such verbs are irregularly spelled find a rule! Point out,

for example, that what remains unchanged during the inflection[5] of
certain verbs is the consonants, the consonant sequence, and what
is modified is the vowels. With this you give him something tangible.
Indicate that so far as the basic structure (and also the "meaning")
of many of the most commonly used verbs is concerned, it is the consonants that count more. Then immediately offer a cluster of words
to substantiate the "rule" you have found. Here are some examples:

FIGHT	FOUGHT
WRITE	WROTE
SPEAK	SPOKE
FIND	FOUND
RING	RANG
DRINK	DRANK
STICK	STUCK
SEE	SAW

Don't be afraid of even further generalizations, further "rules."
Don't be afraid of a scholarly attitude. Don't "entertain." Talk seriously about problems in linguistics. Children are clever enough to
understand. They don't have to be bothered with suburban, nonconcept, family interest words in third grade. Teach them rules. Point
out to them that there is a basic difference between the respective
roles vowels and consonants play in structuring words. Teach them,
point out to them, that *consonants always* (well, almost always) *sound
the same.* Emphasize this important rule! A child should realize that
the written or printed symbol R always sounds /r/, the P always
sounds /p/, the M always sounds /m/, in every English word, in fact
in every language which avails itself of the Latin script. Thus, once a
child (whether three or six years old) has learned the sound of the
symbols B and G[6] and the "basic" sound of the five Latin vowels

A   E   I   O   U

and has accepted the imperative that *English words are to be read
from left to right*, there is no reason why he should spend his precious
time memorizing the "word images" (with "meanings") such as

BAG   BEG   BIG   BOG   BUG

when it is so easy to "de-code" them.

There is never anything "irregular" about consonants.[7] It is vowels that offer spelling problems. What teachers or educators call the irregularity, the haphazardness, of English spelling refers almost exclusively to the vowels, to the complex (but in historical terms generally explicable and justifiable) manner in which English spelling "encodes" the variegated English vowel sounds for which no simple written symbols exist.

I don't mean that the teacher should conceal difficulties. English spelling *is* difficult, certainly much more difficult than the spelling of such almost phonetically spelled languages as Czech or Italian. But it is neither haphazard nor irregular, and even the difficulties (with the few exceptions just noted) are restricted to the realm of vowels. The difficulties arose (and the teacher can explain this to a normal class) because English spelling, like Anglo-Saxon civilization, has tried to meet and reconcile several (in themselves contradictory) challenges:

1. It wanted to preserve the historical character of the language, and to indicate the origin of words, even the period of their incorporation into the vernacular.

2. It wanted to indicate (at least to suggest) pronunciation as accurately as possible.

3. It tried to compromise with the continuing changes of the spoken tongue in the course of centuries.

As will be seen, in later chapters I shall repeatedly refer to these contradictory challenges. One has to understand the spelling of English, not condemn it. Only then can he come to love and appreciate the language, and only if one loves and appreciates it can he then teach it effectively.

Let me return to those verbs which allegedly have irregular, haphazard spelling. The teacher might easily discover and present another rule. She might direct the pupil's attention to the fact that verb forms which denote action in the so-called present tense quite often carry an I- or E-related vowel sound. (In the terms used by linguists these are "front" vowel sounds.) She might give some examples:

FIGHT   WRITE   STICK   SPEAK   BREAK
FIND   DRINK   EAT   SEE

In contradistinction, the same verbs, when indicating an action already fulfilled carry sounds represented by A or O or U. (Linguists speak of "back" vowel sounds.) Thus:

FOUGHT	WROTE	STUCK	SPOKE	BROKE[8]
FOUND	DRANK	ATE	SAW	
	(DRUNK)			

Sometimes, rarely, an /ee/-sounding vowel will change into an /e/, as in

BLEED	BLED
BREED	BRED
FLEE	FLED
MEET	MET
READ (present)	READ (past)[9]

Clusters of words useful in teaching any of the rules discovered spring to mind. This is the beauty of phonics, of the "code" technique. As soon as the form of a word fits some rule, one finds other words to follow the same rule. One key always opens many doors. In sad contradistinction, the "meaning" technique teaches *individual* words to be remembered, with no relation to other words. To repeat: It is important for a child to be able to work out, *on his own*, that FIGHT signifies ("de-codes" into) the sound sequence *f-ī-t* and

> FOUGHT signifies ("de-codes" into) the sound sequence *f-aw-t*.[10]

He does not have to be taught what these sound sequences "mean." He "knows" the spoken words. It is the teacher's job to show him how to do the "de-coding." This is what phonics is all about. "Phonics" is not a philosophical doctrine of a psychological system. It is a technique for "en-coding" and especially for "de-coding" words, with emphasis on "de-coding."

Although I constantly try to find "rules" and to emphasize their significance, I am not too worried if the child finds instances in which some rule I have just given him does not hold. I safeguard myself by emphasizing the word "usually." In the examples

BRING	BROUGHT
TELL	TOLD
HOLD	HELD
BITE	BIT

One or the other of the rules just given does not hold. We just have to point out these seeming exceptions and reassure the child that later on we shall find some added or some better fitting rule or rules.[11]

An older child might be interested to know that in the Hebrew language the dependence of meaning on consonant sequence is carried *ad ultimum.* What the English language does with some verbs Hebrew does as a rule, even as a matter of principle. It expresses all kinds of modifications of meaning by a change of vowels, retaining strict consonant structure:

shomer	=	(one) watching,
shamar	=	(he) watched,
eshmor	=	(I shall) watch,
yashmir	=	(he will be) watched,
mishmar	=	a guardhouse,
ashmurah	=	a watch, a guard
shimurim	=	vigils

No one has the feeling that there is anything irregular about this arrangement.

The sequence example HOLD-HELD once taught me an important lesson. Realizing that it contradicts the usual present-past change of vowel (the 0 signifies the present and the E signifies the past) I asked a boy who was a poor reader whether these sentences

> I HOLD a book yesterday
> I HELD a book now

are correct. He answered that they were not correct, that HOLD refers to something done now and HELD means something finished. There was obviously nothing wrong with this boy's understanding of "meaning." What he was poor in was de-coding of symbols.

At the risk of being repetitious (a teacher must be repetitious), I want to stress once more this very important point: Children expect law and order. They need a world that is reasonable. They cannot grow up to be healthy adults without a father image. Much too soon will they find out about the unreasonableness of our life, our wars, our code of ethics, our institutions. We must preserve at least one illusion — the illusion that language, the means of communication, the supreme gift we have received from our ancestors, the supreme gift we can bestow on our children, is reasonable.

Avoid if you can the term "exception." Avoid even more the term "irregular." Remember: A new "rule" is a new key; a new "exception" is a new stumbling block.

NOTES

[1]Authors' estimates range from 2000 to such high figures as to be unlikely.

[2]The main argument for the "meaning" technique is that most of the basic, simple, "family interest" words with which the child is "familiar" are "irregularly" spelled, and that therefore, they have to be memorized visually and individually.

[3]Note that the word "read" carries different meanings (answers to different definitions) for adherents of the two different teaching philosophies.

[4]I don't generally follow any system (e.g., that of *Webster's New International Dictionary*) in syllabizing words. I try to encourage the child to guess the sound of long words by subdividing them in different ways:

NO-MI-NA-TION   NOM-IN-A-TION   etc.

One form or another finally clicks.

[5]I am not, at this time, prepared to make statements about when and how the teacher should introduce the terms (and concepts) "declension" (of nouns) and "conjugation" (of verbs). I am not sure anything is gained by calling the conjugation of certain verbs "strong," at least in the earliest grades of school. I can only intimate how "meaning" and "de-coding" can both, and in best harmony, help to introduce these significant ideas of grammar if they are used skillfully.

[6]The idea that children should learn to read words (and "meaning") before they are taught the alphabet is to my mind so absurd that I must abstain from discussing it. (See Chall, 1967, on this if you are interested.)

[7]The seeming exceptions are C. G. and S (if you want to call them "exceptions"), each of which represents two different sounds, only two sounds, no more. Some consonants have in a few rare combinations lost their sound value. Thus the K in words like KNIGHT and the W in words like WRONG carry on for historic reasons though their sound value has submerged.

[8]Why the /ī/ sound in FIGHT and WRITE, or the /ee/ sound in EAT and SEE, is indicated in two different ways is another matter in need of further analysis. But the role of "front" vowels versus "back" vowels still holds, and is worth knowing.

It is also worth knowing that all these verbs are of Germanic origin, so we can expect to find a similar rule in German. And indeed the shift from "front" to "back" vowel is obvious in the German verbs below:

Present tense	Past tense	Related noun
SINGT (sings)	SANG (sang)	
BRINGT (brings)	BRACHTE (brought)	
BRICHT (breaks)	BRACH (broke)	BRUCH (break)
SPRICHT (speaks)	SPRACH (spoke)	SPRUCH (saying)
DENKT (thinks)	DACHTE (thought)	
FICHT (fights)	FOCHT (fought)	

[9]In this last example the new "rule" holds, although for some reason unknown to me the spelling of the vowel has remained unchanged. We face a similar problem with

HEAR (present)   HEARD (past)

[10]It is too complicated to indicate the individual phonemes in the agreed form all the time; it becomes tiresome to the reader. Instead of spelling out /f/-/ī/-/t/ or /f/-/aw/-/t/, from now on I shall usually write *f-ī-t* or *f-aw-t,* or even *fīt* and *fawt.*

[11]The sequence TELL-TOLD is a good example. It offers an occasion to show that there exists another group of verbs, the past tense of which is formed by adding a D (or ED). The exception, the seeming exception, gives way to an important rule.

CHAPTER THREE

*A Short Primer on Phonics — Retroactive Modifiers —
The Silent E at the End of Words — The Silent E as a
Modifier of C and G — The Silent E of French Ortho-
graphy — Other Retroactive Modifiers — English Spelling
Is Mindful of Word History and Word Origins — Homo-
phones — The Choice of the Proper Modifier — Vowel
Digraphs — English Spelling: A Reliable Guide to Pro-
nunciation*

Teaching reading by a phonics technique offers immediate rewards.
Every new phonic rule gives a child a new key to clusters of new
words. Phonics encourages guessing. It does not stultify it. I encourage parents and teachers to make up such word clusters. Take the
cluster of sample words[1]

HAT   FAT   MAT   RAT

through which the teacher has familiarized the child with the short
and "basic" sound value /a/ of the letter A. Once the child understands the significance of the retroactive silent E, he will readily
transpose these words into words with the long vowel sound /a/, into

HATE   FATE   MATE   RATE

and just as readily add new examples on his own. Once the child has
learned the short and basic sound value of the other four vowel signs
/e/,/i/,/o/, and /u/ in examples like

MET and PET   DOT and NOT
DIM and FIN   CUT and US[2]

he can easily be taught that the silent E transforms these words into words with the respective long vowel sounds /ee/,/i/,/ō/, and /yo͞o/,[3] into

METE and PETE   DOTE and NOTE
DIME and FINE   CUTE and USE

into words with a different (and at the same time *long*) vowel sound. Dozens of word clusters can be collected by parent or teacher around each of these words. The child will have no trouble in guessing correctly. By the way, the words with the silent E

MATE   PETE   FINE   DOTE   CUTE

also give the child the *names* of the five written vowels:

A   E   I   O   U

Indeed, the significance of the concept silent E is tremendous. After a child has mastered the sounds of the consonants (as I said, they show little variation) and the basic sounds of the five written vowels and has practiced clusters of words around every one of these vowels, the immediate next step is to familiarize him with the role of the silent E. With this, I introduce the concept of retroactive vowel modification and teach a child to exercise retroactive attention. *Without these concepts clear in his mind, a child cannot ever learn to spell English!*

There is much to be learned about the English language just through the example of this single modifier. Here are two rules to teach:

(a) *The silent E is generally the last letter in the word in which it acts.*[4]

(b) *The silent E is seldom farther than two phonemes from the vowel it modifies.*

In the examples

LIE   PIE   TIE
DOE   FOE   HOE   ROE   (GO!)[5]
BLUE   CLUE   (HUE)   TRUE

the silent E follows the vowel to be modified immediately; in

HERE	MERE			
LIFE	PIPE	PIKE		
DOLE	HOLE	MORE	FORE	SHORE
RULE	CHUTE	(CUTE)	(USE)[6]	

it is in its familiar and most common place; and in a few instances like

HASTE   PASTE   TASTE

it acts as far back as the vowel three phonemes removed. This, however, is the exception.

In examples like

FARCE   FORCE   FORGE   PRINCE   FRINGE
HINGE   RIDGE   BRIDGE   (MORGUE!)

the modifying effect upon the vowel is lost, however. The E is just too far from the vowel.

These last examples were so chosen as to introduce a secondary, though significant, modifying effect of the letter E, a retroactive effect upon the pronunciation of the preceding consonants C and G. Usually, C sounds like /k/ and G sounds like /g/ as in the common words

CAT or CAR
GUN or RAG

But either an E or an I changes the sound value of these letters. A child must soon learn the following rules:

(a) *When C is followed by E or I, it sounds like /s/.*

(b) *When G is followed by E or I, it usually (not always!) sounds like /j/.*

In words like those given in the cluster of examples above, the E is the last letter and remains silent. But it retains its sound value if it follows a C or G and is not the last letter. The I, on the other hand, never loses its sound. It is never silent. Here are some examples:

GUN GAME GEM GIN GIST (GET!) (GIVE!) (GILT!) (GILL!)
CAT COT CUT CAPE CENT CIST CITE

(In the last word the I modifies the C while being itself modified by a silent E.)

In the following cluster of words,

LACE CAGE PACE PAGE RACE RAGE DICE RICE

the silent E figures as a double modifier, affecting both the vowel and the preceding consonant, while in examples like

CENTRE (the somewhat affected English spelling)

the E is not really silent. The American spelling

CENTER

properly pushes the E into its correct position.

The following cluster of words, while admittedly somewhat out of context, is best introduced at this point:

BACK/BAKE
DICK/DIKE
LICK/LIKE
PECK
PICK/PIKE
TICK (TIC!)
DOCK
POCK/POKE
DUCK/DUKE

These examples show that the shortness of the basic vowel sound can also be quasi-retroactively indicated. This is done by doubling the consonant that follows the vowel. In the special case of the /k/ sound, this is accomplished by spelling the double letter as CK, in the old Germanic way. Other examples for this rule are:

FELL   FULL
HELL   HILL   HULL
DIG/DIG-GING
FIT/FIT-TER

while

FALL   HALL   ODD

show that the rule does not always strictly hold. In these words the vowel is not truly short. Such items are best memorized.[7]

As a last example for a modified C or G I like to give

CAN-CEL   GAGE (or GAUGE)

They are just examples to show a child both possible pronunciations of C or G in a single word.

Always present a child with clusters of examples. This makes word solving a routine procedure. Never repeat the same words in stories, the way the look-and-say technique recommends. Teaching reading is *not* teaching the meaning of words. Even the most severely dyslexic boy will understand most of the words I have used in these examples when they are sounded to him. He does not have to be taught their meaning. What he has to practice is "de-coding" them.

There is one more minor and not too common role to the silent E. The originators of English spelling seem to have abhorred a letter S at the end of words. (They probably felt that the S ending must retain its character as a sign of the *plural* or the *possessive*. Thus, if the morpheme ends in an /s/ we must add a silent E to the phonogram, a kind of E *à la française* that becomes a sounded E when pronunciation so requires.

HORSE (HORSES/HORSE'S)
HOUSE   MOUSE
GOOSE (GEESE!)   MOOSE

are some examples. There are a few exceptions, among them

LENS/LENSES

a Latin-derived word which is reluctantly used by the public as a *singular*. My patients often tell me that their LENS ARE dirty, while some have written that their left LENSE is broken.

Some of these words with that E *à la française* also sport "irregular" plural forms, like

LOUSE   LICE
MOUSE   MICE
(DIE!)   DICE

In these plurals the silent E figures in both of its modifying actions: it modifies the I *and* the C. However, there are words of similar ending,

POLICE   CAPRICE
CHALICE   MALICE
PRACTICE

in which the E is purely a modifier for the sound value of the C and does not modify the sound of the I. The reason was not altogether clear to me until I noted that the examples just given are all dissyllables and apparently non-Anglo-Saxon. They are, in fact, later, French-influenced, not yet fully assimilated acquisitions of the English language whereas LICE and MICE are older Germanic words. It seems that only in the Anglo-Saxon, not in the French-derived words, will the E modify the I of the ending -ICE. Remembering the double modifying effect of the silent E in

LACE   MACE   RACE   GRACE
PAGE   RAGE

words like

GRIMACE   PALACE   SOLACE
BARRAGE   GARAGE   MIRAGE
(COURAGE[8] RUMMAGE   SHORTAGE)

offer a similar problem, and answer to the same explanation: the silent E at the end of a word plays a somewhat different role in still-foreign French-origin words and in words that are English to begin with or have been totally Anglicized. It is *not* because English spelling and pronunciation know no rules that in

LICE and POLICE
LACE and PALACE
RAGE and GARAGE

the modifying effect of the silent E is different. With care and interest one can find the rationale behind these differences. And I don't think that a child in third grade is too immature to be taught some of the history of the English language and be given such rationales.

I started my discussion of the retroactive modifiers with the French word

HÂTE

I noted that the fourth character, the silent E (which to the French indicates that the third grapheme, the T, is to be pronounced), is not essentially a sound symbol but a pronunciation guide, so much so that it could be just as well replaced by some other directive sign (not necessarily a letter) should French consensus so decide.[9] The silent E of French spelling appears to me a kind of prototype of retroactive modifiers, and I would not be surprised if historians of English spelling found it the model for later English adoption.

I feel that a few remarks about the French version of this modifier will not be out of place in our present context, that in fact they might clarify some points.

Dropping of consonants (especially of crowding consonants, but also of certain solitary consonants) is very much among the characteristics of spoken French, and special reminders are therefore needed to keep such consonants sounded. In the word

TARD (pronounced /t/-/āh/-/r/)

the last letter is silent, and its presence in the written word can be understood only if we look at the word's history. It derives from the Latin

TARDUS (TARDE)

Even if not pronounced, the D is part of the word's "consonant frame." When the grapheme D *is* to be pronounced, a retroactive sign (I emphasize: a sign, not a symbol) becomes a necessity. Thus, the word

GARDE (pronounced /g/-/āh/-/r/-/d/)

sports a silent terminal E which, in French spelling, always acts upon the *immediately preceding* letter symbol, *which is a consonant.* Whatever the historic relationship between the French silent E and the English silent E, they don't have the same functional significance in the two languages. In the French version the silent E (and here I refer only to the silent E that concludes a word) acts upon a *consonant;* in the English version it modifies the sound value of a *vowel.*

Nor is this the only modifying role of the letter E in French spelling. Just as in English, C and G are retroactively modified by the letter E (also by I). In fact, in this respect, English, a Germanic language, is much in line with Romance languages: the letters E and I modify the sound of C and G in every one of them. In this second of its modifying roles the E is not necessarily at the end of the word and, just as in English, it is now always silent. A few examples must suffice. In

FORCE	TIGE	CEINTURE
MORCEAU	GEAI	JEAN

the E is silent while in

$$\text{CENTIME} \quad \text{CERCEAU} \quad \text{CÉRÉALE}$$
$$\text{GENTIL} \quad \text{GERME} \quad \text{GERANT} \quad \text{LEGÈRE}$$

the E retains full vowel character. The examples have been chosen to show that an E which follows a C or G can retain its modifying influence upon these consonants whatever its pronunciation. (There are two C-modifying E's in CERCEAU, with only one of them pronounced.) Note also that in

$$\text{CAISSON}$$

the sound of the C is unmodified though the vowel digraph which follows the letter sounds very much like the English /e/.[10]

The similarity between the French and English handling of at least certain spelling problems extends, we may add, even to the use of what we might best call a de-modifier. In the French words

$$\text{VOGUE} \quad \text{GUERRE} \quad \text{GUIGNOL}$$

and in the English words

$$\text{GUEST} \quad \text{GUIDE}$$

the G sound remains unmodified by the following E or I sound. (In the case of VOGUE the E remains silent.) An intercalated pronunciation guide, a silent de-modifier (it takes the form of a U) indicates the cancellation of the modifying action of the E or I. Why in words like

$$\text{GARÇON}$$

the modifying is done by a *cedilla* rather than with a silent E, I don't really know. My knowledge of French is too fragmentary for that.

The next steps in teaching phonics lead further into the depths of English spelling. There are more of those retroactive modifiers or, more precisely, retroactive vowel sound modifiers. They are less frequently encountered than the silent E, and they are more difficult to master. I shall mention only a few of them, the modifying W, the modifying GH, the sundry modifiers of the vowel I and the modifying R, and I think we shall do best by always returning to the basic sound value of individual vowels as a starting point. Here are some instances: Our pupils have become familiar with the basic sound of A, E, and O in words like

$$\text{SAP and RAP} \quad \text{PET and FED} \quad \text{LOT and ROD}$$

They must now learn that a W retroactively modifies the sound of these vowels into /aw/, /yo͞o/, and /o͞/ respectively, e.g.,

SAW and RAW   PEW and FEW   LOW and ROW

Our pupils learned about the basic sound value of the letter I in words like

THIN   FIT   LIT
KIN and KID   FIN and SIN
CHILL and WILL

and about the modifying effect of the silent E; they must now learn that the letter groups GH, ND, NT, GN, LD modify the basic I sound into /ī/ in a similar manner.

THIGH   FIGHT   LIGHT
KIND   BIND   BLIND
PINT and SIGN
CHILD   MILD   WILD

are some good examples to memorize. Our pupils will also know how to pronounce such simple words (with basic vowels sounds) as

HEN   FIN   FUN   RUN

They must learn that *if it is an R that follows these vowels*, then the vowel sound usually changes and in a rather peculiar manner. Thus

HER sounds *hûr*
FIR and FUR sound *fûr*
URN sounds *ûrn*

Words like

FIRE   HIRE   TIRE   WIRE

offer some added peculiarities, as if both the R that follows the letter I and the silent E that ends the word compete to modify the stem vowel. In the end, the I sounds /ĭ/, the sound being followed by a kind of short and aborted /ûr/. It almost sounds like *fĭ-ûr*.

Words that contain an O followed by R offer some problems. In some of them

FOR   FORD   FORK   FORM   FORT
SHORT   SPORT   YORK

the R seems to act rather meekly, while in others

WORD   WORK   WORM   WORTH

the vowel once more changes to /ûr/. The teacher might at this time point out to the student that retroactive modifiers are, obviously, not always silent. Although in the words

RATE   BITE   FIGHT   SAW   ROW

the retroactive modifiers are not themselves phonemes (they are just unpronounced modifiers), in

KIND   BIND   etc.

and in all the examples in which an R figures, the modifier or modifiers are also pronounced.

The modifying effect of the letter (or sound) R upon the vowel A is no less intriguing. The words

BAR   CAR   FAR   MAR   PAR   (WAR!)

carry a modified vowel sound /äh/ different from the /a/ of HAT, the /ā/ of HATE, and the /āw/ of RAW. The silent E then further complicates matters. We pronounce

BARE   CARE   FARE   MARE   PARE   WARE   (ARE!)

with a vowel /ä/ that is different from the vowel in HATE. Our sound sign A is now quasi-doubly modified. With such examples even a child can learn, and quite early in his learning career, that an A, for example, can be pronounced in at least five different ways.[11] This will not confuse him in the least. Safely guided by the different modifiers, the child will proceed with assurance. He will confidently guess what sound to utter. Indeed, the phonic method gives wings to teaching and learning while presentation in clusters provides the solid foundation efficient reading is so much in need of.

After the teacher has collected and presented clusters of words with the A-plus-W and the A-plus-R combination, she might find it opportune to introduce the combination A-plus-L at this juncture, since the L in this combination sometimes also acts as a modifier of sorts. To be sure, the L will do this only when crowded out by certain other consonants. Also, although it affects the sound value of the preceding A, it will itself often be barely audible. Here are three sets of examples:

(1) TALK, WALK, STALK (A sounds /aw/, L hardly audible).
(2) BALD, BALL, TALL, WALL (A sounds /aw/, L well pronounced).
(3) BALM, CALM, PALM (A sounds /āh/, L hardly audible).
In the first two clusters the vowel is similar to that in

LAW   RAW   SAW
CLAW   BRAWL   BRAWN

In the third the vowel sounds like that in

CAR   CARD   FAR   FARM   HARM
START   (WAR   WARD   WARM!)

There is still another letter combination, S-plus-T, that affects the pronunciation of the preceding A. Again the best way to familiarize a child with this modifier is through clusters of words like

CAST   LAST   PAST   (PASTE!)
VAST   (WASTE!)

and "combination clusters" like

BAR   BALM   BLAST   (BARE!)
CAR   CALM   CAST   (CARE!)
FAR   FARM   FAST   (FARE!)
MAR   MART   MAST   (MARE!)

which are as good an aid for memorizing rules as any the teacher can wish.

Once the child has sufficiently grown up to ask "Why?" or "How come?" merely emphasizing agreement as a basis for spelling will not do as an answer. *English is a highbrow language.* One needs a dictionary truly to savor it. Take the words

CERTAIN   SERVE   SURF
FIRM   CURVE   WORD

The modified vowel-plus-R sound is the same in all six (= /ûr/), and the first phoneme (= /s/) is identical in the first three. Why, then, the variegation? Only the dictionary will tell the child that the last word is Germanic and that its German cognate, WORT, is spelled with an O whereas four of the other five examples derive from the Latin (the origin of SURF is "unknown," according to Webster), their roots in Latin being

CERT-   SERV-   FIRM-   CURV-

respectively. We must have agreement on both spelling and sound, but only history explains their sometimes strange-looking bonds. We must not be afraid to use a dictionary; one cannot start teaching its use early enough. We must tell our pupils about the origins of English words as soon as possible, as soon as they can ask questions. Let us not clutter a child's mind, let us not waste his precious time with artless and uninteresting stories about Tim and Sally and the dog, repeating the same words dozens of times!

Here are more examples:

FIN   FINE
FIT   FIGHT
SIN   SIGN

Is it absurd or illogical, is it unnecessarily complicating English spelling to use three different kinds of retroactive modifiers (the silent E in one case, the silent GH in the second, and the silent G in the third) all to achieve the same end, to modify the sound of the I? Or to put it into a still simpler form: Why bother with letter groups

-INE   -IGN
-ITE   -IGHT

to signify the same sounds? The answer can be given only in terms of history. Why not tell the child about that history? Children are not stupid, and English is a tongue to challenge the intellect. One cannot learn to spell the language by playing in school, by listening to stories, or by looking at pictures. We must teach etymology; we must teach word history. First of all, of course, we must teach the phonic rules of pronunciation and spelling. The child knows what the meaning is of

fĭn   fĭt   sĭn

when he hears the words. He does not have to be taught their meaning. He also does not have to see the words

FINE   FIGHT   SIGN

repeated in banal stories until he has acquired a "visual image" of
them, a "visual image attached to meaning." Phonics will teach him
how to pronounce the words using the rules of retroactive modification, and once he has pronounced them, he will know that he knows
them. But finally he should know why they are spelled the way they
are, and why in any particular case one particular modifier is used
and not another. Why is one modifier used in FINE, another in
FIGHT ("Why don't we write FITE?"), and still another in SIGN?
We owe the child an answer. To refer to "agreement" is not sufficient. We can, of course, just present him with a "rule": "FIGHT is
spelled with the silent GH as vowel modifier. It is 'incorrect' to spell
it FITE." But this will not do for long. We had better try to justify
and explain the choice in terms of the history of the individual words.

I want to elaborate on this feature of English spelling, one of its
most attractive aspects. I have for this purpose chosen an assortment
of homophones. I hope that through these examples I can elucidate
some of the rules by which retroactive modifiers came to be utilized
(also some other spelling props) and also clarify the significance of
English spelling peculiarities as a means to meaning. These examples should at the same time typify the essentially historical basis of
English spelling and its logic. The four homophones of my first example are

RITE   RIGHT   WRITE   WRIGHT

The first word, RITE, has to do with the conduct of religious
ceremonies, and obviously derives from the Latin word RITUS, of
which only the first three letters, the root, were retained, though with
lengthening of the center vowel. The simplest of all retroactive modifiers, the silent E, indicates this.

The second word is more peculiarly spelled, at least for those
who know no other language but English and also don't understand
the spirit of its script. There is nothing peculiar or absurd (these are
epithets one often finds attached to English spelling) in the spelling of
this word, and those who know German will already have realized
that the word is cognate with the German RECHT.[12] What happened
is obvious: the original guttural /kh/ got lost in spoken English, but
its symbol equivalent, GH, was retained and turned into a retroactive
determinant of the sounded quality of the written I. It is in the
spirit of "Anglo-Saxon" thinking and speaking to change the sound

but retain the form. To keep new wine in old bottles, a Labor government sworn in by a Queen, is very much a British characteristic. English spelling simply turned the GH digraph into a determinant (or modifier) which indicates that the sounded I is long.

The third of our homophones is WRITE, a word cognate with the German REISSEN (= to draw), by now a rare word, which those who went to a German school will remember from words like REISS-BRETT or REISSZEUG.[13] In old German the word started with a W sound (perhaps sounded like WREISS) which both the English and the Germans dropped from pronunciation, but which the English, characteristically, kept in their spelling.

The fourth word, WRIGHT, is, of course, also of Germanic origin. English *is* a Germanic language. Its cognate in German is WIRKEN, "to work," or RICHTEN, one meaning of which is "to repair." Both the old Germanic W and the old Germanic CH (for centuries CH and GH were interchangeable) were retained in the English written word.

The beauty of all this is in its logic. One can be sure that RITE does not apply to my right hand or the act I perform when I put these words onto paper. Nor does it signify the man who repairs my boat or cart. *Both logic and a sense of history permeate English spelling.*

Let us not complain abouts its hopeless and confusing "irregularities." There is rarely anything irregular or haphazard about English spelling. It is almost always logically contrived, and its foundation lies in history. Take the words

CITE   SITE   SIGHT

as another attractive example. The first word is the anglicized form of the Latin CITARE, the second of the Latin SITUS (with the silent E to indicate the pronunciation of the I in both of them), and the last is cognate with the German SICHT. One can again be sure that the "ideogram" SITE is not the synonym of "vision" and that SIGHT is never a reference to a "location." Nor will it ever mean the calling of someone to court.

I could go on multiplying examples like these, one more interesting, more convincing, than the other. Homophones such as

SINE (from SINUS) and SIGN (from SIGNUM)

hardly need an explanation of the proper choice of retroactive modifiers for those with some knowledge of Latin, from which both of these words derive.

A most interesting pair of homophones is

NIGHT   KNIGHT

We may expect that both words have Germanic cognates, the first in the German NACHT, the other in the German KNECHT. Again there is nothing arbitrary, in fact there is history and logic, in the assignment of meaning to these homophones. One can be sure that KNIGHT is not an ideogram denoting the antonym of DAY. The "ideogram" KNIGHT gives us, by the way, a key to the understanding of a whole series of other seemingly peculiar spellings: KNEE, KNOT, KNEAD, and KNOW, with their German cognates, KNIE, KNOTEN, KNETEN, and KENNEN, giving away the historical reason for the presence of that strange K (a veritable rudiment) in the spelled word. And again, if we pick the interesting homophones

NAVE   KNAVE

there can be no question that it is the first "ideogram" that signifies the center hall of a church, deriving as it does from the Latin NAVIS, whereas the second, earmarked as Germanic by the first two letters, comes from a word that is KNABE in present day German. Let me repeat, English written words have not ceased to be phonograms of spoken words. A written English word may acquire, will acquire, for the advanced reader, certain characteristics of ideograms (he looks at KNAVE and knows what it means) but it never is an ideogram in the sense in which ੪ meant an ox or ♯ meant a fence in old Semitic writing, and especially not in the sense in which the notation $6 + 4 = 10$ does. NAVE and KNAVE are still, and primarily, *ordered sequences of sound symbols.* Both display the same modifier (a silent E); the second also has K added — a prop for easier identification with meaning.

The English morphemes (they are identical) which these two written words symbolize both start with /n/ and end in /v/. In an appropriate sequence, both written words contain a symbol for /n/ more *to the left* and a symbol for /v/ more *toward the right.* (That silent E, the retroactive determinant, is, as I have said, added only to indicate the proper pronunciation of the vowel sign A.) Thus, NAVE and KNAVE are phonograms first of all. But in addition (note: in addition) the *seen* word forms are imbued with meaning. This is the unique beauty of written English. George Bernard Shaw's invectives against written English seem to me downright silly.

The following sets of homophones will serve to introduce the concept of digraphs — two letters representing one sound; in these particular examples, two vowel signs representing one vowel sound. (Only the latter necessitates discussion. Consonant digraphs like TH, CH, SH offer as few phonic problems as consonants in general.) Homophones with vowel digraphs make up a considerable corpus of English words, and we are often told that the spelling differences, the use of different vowel digraphs for the same phoneme, serve the purpose of differentiating them visually through a look-and-see-meaning approach. But while this is true, it certainly is not a sufficient explanation.

Let us look at the homophones

VANE   VAIN   VEIN

three different spellings of the same morpheme (one making use of the familiar retroactive silent E, and each of the other two employing a different digraph) with three different meanings. Have the different spellings been assigned respective meanings according to the whim of some Doctor Johnson? Certainly not. Again there is history behind each choice. There was, in fact, no choice. Looking at the word VANE with the linguist's eye, we realize that the word is a cognate of the German FAHNE (a "flag") while VAIN (think also of the Latin-derived word VANITY) is a French word and VEIN is the anglicized form of the Latin VENA (a "conduit").

Quite interesting are the homophones,

RAIN   REIN   REIGN

The first is an obvious cognate of the German REGEN (it lost the consonant G along its way), the second word comes from the French, and the third derives from the Latin REGNUM. In the last word the sound of the "crowding" G is lost but the written consonant is retained. "English cussedness or conservatism," we may say. But we can also add, "English utilitarianism." The letter does visually separate REIN from REIGN.[14]

There is no point in crowding the examples. In these two sets we have met with the equal-sounding vowel digraphs

AI   EI

and will make a mental note that both sound /ā/. We shall also always (or in most cases) expect to find some historical reason why one or the other has been assigned to its respective meaning.

As an example of another pair of equal-sounding vowel digraphs we note

IE   EA

In the homophones

PIECE   PEACE

the respective digraphs both sound like /ee/ and the silent E merely indicates that the letter C is to be pronounced /s/. They are "French" not "English" silent E's! The first word is a simple transliteration of the French PIÈCE; the second carries the A of the Latin PAX and the French PAIX. In the homophone pair

ATE   EIGHT

one of the members carries the modifying silent E and the vowel sound, of course, is /ā/. There cannot be any question which of the two homophones signifies the numeral 8 if we remember that ACHT is the German cognate for the numeral.

I should now like to discuss the problem of vowel digraphs more systematically. Admittedly, it is one of the most challenging problems in the phonics approach to teaching a child to read. But first a short digression is in order.

Having tried to convince my readers of the logic, even beauty, of English spelling in terms of history (etymology), I should be permitted to show that, with modifiers and digraphs which are supposedly so confusing, English spelling actually is a highly reliable and logical guide to pronunciation. Statements to the contrary abound. I think that such statements show nothing but a lack of understanding of the rules that govern both of them. There are, of course, exceptions. But they are exceptions.

Let me give a few examples, rather simple examples. They were so chosen that all that proper pronunciation requires is awareness of the principle of retroactive modification and some familiarity with the rules of the silent E, the modifying R, and the modified G, all discussed earlier. The silent E, e.g., the one that concludes the words

RATE   RIDE

clearly indicates that the A sounds /ā/ and the I sounds /ī/. There is nothing equivocal, nothing haphazard. No other pronunciation is even imaginable. One just has to be aware of the rule of the silent E. In the words

RACE   RICE

the concluding silent E also, and unequivocally, indicates that the letter C must be pronounced as /s/. The spelling rules out any confusion with RAKE, RAZE, RASE, or RISE, which are all different words with different meanings. Words like

FAR   MAR   PAR   SCAR   LARK   PART

must (the R indicates this) be pronounced with an /āh/ sound, while in

FARE, FAIR(!)   HARE, HAIR(!)   PARE, PAIR(!)
RARE   SCARE   SPARE   STARE, STAIR(!)

the vowel sound is /ä/. No confusion, no alternative.

No doubt we ought to make some concession here to the look-and-say technique. In the cluster of examples just given, FARE and FAIR, HARE and HAIR, PARE and PAIR, and also STARE and STAIR are homophones and, as I indicated earlier, it is the appearance of the words, the spelling of the homophones, that give away the meaning. But as far as pronunciation is concerned, there is nothing equivocal. Complicated as it may appear, a child must learn that the digraph AI, when followed by R, stands for the same vowel sound (/ä/) as the letter A does when followed by R *and* the silent E. Thus, in pronunciation.

FARE = FAIR HARE = HAIR PARE = PAIR STARE = STAIR[15]

The child also has to learn that whenever an R is not involved, AI stands for the long sound /ā/. The example VANE = VAIN = VEIN was given earlier. A few further examples are here best presented with their homophones:

LAIN, LANE   MAIN, MANE   PAIL, PALE   PAIN, PANE

I am not aware of any exceptions.

To show the adequacy (in most cases, anyway) of English spelling to indicate the sound of English words, I might now turn to a different group of examples — one already discussed. In

GIN   GEM   WAGE

the E or I modifies the sound value of the preceding G, while in the last word the concluding E also continues in its terminal modifying role. In the examples

GUEST (GHETTO!)   GUILD   VAGUE   GUIDE

the modifying value of the E or I is undone, while in the last two words the silent E continues in its typical act. The student just has to learn about the existence of a de-modifying silent U (or H) once and for all.[16] We are confronted with rules. No mistake in pronunciation is possible.

In words like

HORSE   RAISE

the silent E is purely cosmetic, not a modifier. One has to know that this is one of its multiple roles. Neither the O nor the AI are in any way affected.

To demonstrate the logic of spelling, the keys spelling offers for proper pronunciation, the teacher should avail herself of clusters of simple words, such as the following (the first word is the guide word, the "prompter" word):

RID: RIDE, BRIDE   RIDES, BRIDE'S   RIDGE, BRIDGE
         RIDGES, BRIDGET, BRIDGET'S

All of these words are governed by the modifying E in its different roles, silent at times, sounded at others, but always following some simple rules, best learned through these types of examples, freely made up as the teacher proceeds.

The trend in English spelling toward maximum possible accuracy in indicating pronunciation is well demonstrated in another, more sophisticated example:

PEACE   APPEASE

While it is obvious that the two words have the same root and related meanings, it so happens that in spoken and in listened-to language the first word ends in the sound /s/ and the second in the sound /z/. There can never be any argument about pronunciation. The noun PEACE *is* pronounced with an /s/, the verb APPEASE *is* pronounced with a /z/, and that's that. The written word should indicate this fact. And it does. I cannot reiterate often enough, in opposition to "silent" reading, "meaning" reading, "look-and-say" reading, that written words stand for spoken words and read words stand for heard words, and that the primary job of written words and read words is to be symbols of spoken and heard words.

One of my favorite examples for the intrinsic logic of spelling as indicator of pronunciation is the word cluster

FAR   SPAR   SPARE
PAIR   PARE
SPARSE   FARCE

In the first two words the R modifies the sound of A to /äh/. In the third word the concluding RE changes the sound of the A to /ä/. For the next two words we have our ARE = AIR rule. All this follows the guidelines we have already established for the modifying R, the silent E, and the digraph AI. In the last two words the A once more sounds like /äh/. Is this against rules, against the logic of spelling, against expectation? Not at all! The concluding E in SPARSE is only for looks, while in FARCE it serves to define the sound of the C. In each of the two words the A is too far away from the E to be modified by it. Thus, in SPARSE and FARCE the A sounds the way it does in SPAR and FAR and *not* the way it sounds in SPARE and FARE.[17]

NOTES

¹We shall assume from now on that a child has already learned that reading progresses from left to right.

²The letter U offers some difficulties. Less frequently, in words like

PUT   FULL   PULL

the same letter signifies a different short sound, a sound /ŏŏ/, no less "basic."

³Here again, the letter U offers some difficulties. The silent E can also transform the sound into /ōō/.

⁴The child should be taught early that the S of the plural and the 'S of the genitive don't negate this rule. The S of MATES or MATE'S does not change the modifying effect of the E.

⁵I have used parentheses or an exclamation mark (sometimes both), to make the reader aware of some exception or some feature not discussed at the moment. The teacher can always use the opportunity to branch off in a different direction on any of these items.

⁶These examples, mentioned earlier, should give the teacher the opportunity to indicate that there are two alternatives in dealing with the long U. A certain amount of guessing must be encouraged. If /k/-/ōō/-/t/ does not ring a bell, /k/-/yōō/-/t/ probably will.

⁷Originally the vowel *was* short, and in the cognate German words *(Fall, Halle, Ort)* still is. The English changed pronunciation *(consensus!)*, while the spelling remained unchanged *(history!)*.

⁸The word

COURAGE

is an excellent example of the interplay of *pronunciation* and *spelling* in the development of English words. The pronunciation is

kuridj

(with the accent on the first syllable) and about this there can be no argument *(consensus!)*. The word was taken over from the French and remained French in its spelled form *(history!)*. The Germans also adopted the word but, characteristically, changed neither spelling nor pronunciation. Both French and Germans pronounce the word as

koorāhzh

with the accent on the last syllable.

⁹Its role reminds me of the "determinatives" of ancient scripts "placed before or after words . . . not themselves pronounced" (Diringer, 1962). They served as indicators of meaning when some symbol did not give unequivocal information. That it is a vowel, not a consonant, that French orthography singled out for such an auxiliary role is itself to be noted. Consonants are, in general, the structural elements of words, part of their frame, while modification is a job mostly left to vowels and E is the most expendable of all vowels. In the three French words

JEANNE D(E) ARC

the E gives up three chances to be heard, for three different reasons.

[10]Obviously, the French too are history-minded people. The word CAISSON comes from the Italian CASSA; it retains both the /k/ sound and the A in the spelling.

[11]In *Webster's New International Dictionary*, Second Edition (unabridged), there are actually eight sound variants for the letter A.

[12]The only Germanic language I know well is German, more accurately, High German. It is therefore natural for me to refer to the High German cognates of English words whenever the need arises. (Some examples were given earlier.) Other authors might use Dutch or Danish or, especially, Low German examples, which generally are much closer to the English. I must be forgiven; I am not a philologist.

[13]The Hungarian word (the noun) for DRAWING is RAJZ (it rhymes, more or less, with NOISE); it derives from the same root.

[14]The homophones just analyzed offer the teacher a good occasion to introduce an important topic: a discussion of the layered structure of the English vocabulary. Usually one of a pair of homophones will be a more ancient Germanic (Anglo-Saxon) word, and the other Latin-French or Latin. It was the usage of centuries that finally polished words with different meanings into sounded twins. It is the differences in spelling that point out the differences in their origins — RIGHT, SIGHT, KNAVE, VANE, RAIN are Germanic; RITE, CITE, NAVE, VAIN, REIGN are Latin or Latin-French. (The layered structure of English will be discussed further in the chapters that follow.)

[15]There is one obvious exception:

ARE

is not pronounce the way AIR is but the auxiliary verb, (to) BE, is one we really cannot call "regular." Spelling and pronunciation of its variegated forms are best learned by the look-and-say technique. The fact is that *the older a word, the greater the chances of some irregularity.* And the same holds, the more common the word. Certainly, (to) BE is as old and as ubiquitous as words can be. We cannot in its case expect that all rules will be followed.

[16]Why GHASTLY and GHOST contain an H, I cannot explain.

[17]Actually, the two consonants which follow the A in SPARSE and FARCE make their vowels sound shorter. Thus /ăh/ rather than /āh/ is the correct indication of the sound. I shall not be too meticulous in indicating such small differences.

CHAPTER FOUR

Once More: Vowel Digraphs and Homophones — The Schizophrenia of English Spelling — The Letter Y — The Place of the Accent in Two-Syllable Words — A Note on Prefixes and Suffixes — Some Strange Spellings — Homographs

English writing cannot help relying on determinant signs (retroactive modifiers) and on digraphs, to which we now turn, since the language has about 40 sounds but its essentially Latin alphabet consists of only 26 letters. Of course, other languages are faced with the same problem. As far as I can tell, all European spoken languages operate with more than 26 sounds.

Some orthographies made it rather simple, Hungarian, for instance. By applying diacritical marks to the five Latin vowels it created additional signs for vowels of definite *timbre* and duration (= prosodic value) which can easily be learned and do not change the purely phonetic character of the writing. Thus, in Hungarian,

A = /short aw/
Á = /long āh/
É = /long ā/
O = /short o/
Ó = /long ow of ROW/
Ö = /short French eu/
Ő = /long French eu of BLEU/

and so on. The most commonly used vowel, E, is an exception worth mentioning inasmuch as there are actually two distinctly different sounds (an open /a/ and a closed /e/) which Hungarian orthography spells with the same letter E. The degree of difference between the two sounds is different in different regions of Hungary, and I can

still flabbergast (à la Shaw's Professor Higgins) some of my Hungarian patients by telling them what county in Hungary they hail from just by listening to their "open" and
"closed" /e/'s.[1]

Hungarian knows no vowel digraphs, but it has a number of
consonant digraphs. They stand for consonant sounds not covered
by any letter of the Latin alphabet, e.g.,

CS = /ch/   SZ = /s in RICE/   ZS = /zh/

Czech (or Slovak) spelling solved these problems even more
economically. When reading Czech, there is hardly ever any need for
the eye to stop and reconsider the previous letter. The Czechs made
up letters with diacritical signs for consonant sounds or diphthongs
not covered by the Latin alphabet. Among these are

Č = /ch/   Ž = /zh/   Š = /sh/
Ň = /Spanish ñ/   Ř = /rzh/

An occasional digraph, like CH for /kh/, does not complicate
their superbly simple spelling too much.

English spelling makes use of digraphs for some of the same
consonants (CH and SH), and also for two other consonants (the TH
of THIN and the TH of THEN) and a diphthong (the WH of WHEN),
none of them represented in the Latin alphabet. I will only refer to
them briefly. In my teaching method they are also introduced in
clusters, step by step, going from the known to the not-yet-known,
with repetitions of the known, with retroactive modifiers interspersed
for practice purposes. The approach is strictly and definitely phonic.
No story. No "widening of horizon."[2] Some examples are

COP CHOP CHAP HAT CHAT CHIN
CUT HUT SHUT SHIP SHOP SHAPE HARE SHARE
SHINE SHAWL SHREW SHREWD WISH WASH
PAT PATH BATH BATHE NOT MOTH BOTH THIN
THINK THIGH THROW
TAT THAT THEN THERE THIS THE
WET WHET WHAT WHEN WIT WHITE (WHO!)

The great phonic problem of English spelling is vowel digraphs.
To teach the sound value of individual vowel digraphs is not actually

difficult. As a kind of introduction I tell students that, in general, vowel digraphs stand for long vowel sounds for which there is no unequivocal single vowel symbol in our alphabet. I also reassure them by telling them that, again in general, the sound value of vowel digraphs shows little variance, that there are usually no more than one or two ways one can sound some individual digraph. There is no point in frightening students with "haphazardness." Students will prefer a rule, any rule, however vague to haphazardness.

Here are some vowel digraphs and their usual sound values:

EE = /ee/
IE = /ee/ or /ī/[3]
OO = /oo/
OA = /ō/
OE = /ō/
OW = /ō/[4]

Mentioned earlier were

AI = /ā/ (but /ä/ before R)
EI = /ā/ or /ee/ or /ĭ/

OU is only rarely a digraph.[5] In most cases it is nearer a diphthong and sounds like the diphthong in the German HAUBE. Occasionally, as will be seen later, the OW digraph does the same.

One of the difficulties, admittedly, with vowel digraphs is that the sound value of individual digraphs, although relatively constant, is not always the same. As can be gathered from this short list, some digraphs may represent more than one vowel sound. The sound value of the frequently encountered digraph EA is, in fact, almost unpredictable (this being the reason why it was not included in our list). But the true difficulty is superabundance: Which digraph is correct for an /ee/ sound in some individual word? Which digraphs should one use for an /ā/ sound? And when should one use a digraph and when a retroactive modifier to spell a certain vowel sound? As my analysis of the example

VANE   VAIN   VEIN

suggested, the historic-etymologic approach is likely to offer the most plausible answers. But we should not forget *consensus*.

With the following examples, arranged in clusters,

BEER DEER DEEM FEEL KEEL NEED PEEL PEEP PEER SEE
SEED   SEEM   SEEN

FIELD   NIECE   PIECE   PIER   TIER   PIERCE   FIERCE[6]

FOOT[7] LOOP POOL TOOL STOOL SCHOOL ROOM BROOM
(BLOOD!   FLOOD!   FLOOR!)

FOUL LOUD CLOUD PROUD HOUND MOUND POUND ROUND
SOUND   OUT   (SOUL!   SOUR!)

one should, in general, have no difficulties since each cluster represents just one vowel or diphthong sound. Clusters can also be made up, for practice purposes, in a mixed manner, e.g., by pairing different vowel sounds:

FOOL	FOUL
LOOK	LOUD
HOOK	HOUND
STOOP	STOUT

or by pairing different spellings to signify the same vowel sound. (Inventiveness and imagination count for much in the teaching situation.)

For the different spellings in homophones, in the beginning one need not offer anything better than the usual explanation: they help to keep the homophones apart according to meaning. (It would, I must admit, be going too far in a classroom situation to etymologize every single word.) Also, since homophones very often engage a digraph in at least one member of a homophone pair (and more than one in a triplet or quadruplet of homophones) to a beginner a similar answer will also explain the superabundance of vowel digraphs or modifiers. Let us begin with some not too sophisticated examples:

HALE	HAIL	
MALE	MAIL	
SALE	SAIL	
TALE	TAIL	
VALE	VAIL	VEIL
VANE	VAIN	VEIN

HARE	HAIR	(HEIR)
FARE	FAIR	
STARE	STAIR	
ROW	ROE	
TOW	TOE	
SOUL(!)	SOLE	

The digraphs and modifiers in these examples offer little difficulty. The teacher will explain that the AI digraph (also the much less frequently met EI digraph) stands in these examples for the same sound as the A does when it is modified by the silent E. Thus, HAIL sounds like HALE, and VEIL sounds like VALE, and FAIR sounds like FARE. (The modifying character of the R does not get lost.) She might also explain that the modifying (silent) W and the modifying (silent) E both add to the length of the sound /ō/. Thus, ROW and ROE sound the same, but do not look the same or have the same meaning. The solitary example with an OU digraph explains itself.

The English language abounds in homophones. To familiarize a student with the phonics of vowel digraphs, the contrast of homophones offers the best opportunity. Here are some further examples, most of them rather intriguing:

HEART	HART
BREAD	BRED
READ	RED
BEAR	BARE
PEAR	PARE, PAIR
WEAR	WARE
PEAK	PEEK
PEAL	PEEL
READ	REED
SEA	SEE
HEAR	HERE
BREAK	BRAKE
GREAT	GRATE
STEAK	STAKE
SHEAR	SHEER
STEAL	STEEL
WEAK	WEEK
WEAL	WEEL

DEAR	DEER
BEAN	BEEN
BIER	BEER
BEE	BE
BUY	BY (BYE)
DIE	DYE
LIE	LYE
EIGHT	ATE
ROAD	RODE
SOAR	SORE
BOAR	BORE
LOAD	LODE
HOARD	HORDE
TAUGHT	TAUT

Each of these homophones retains its separate meaning despite a different spelling. Why the individual assignments I can in some cases guess but do not, in general, know. Take the first pair of homophones: I do not know why HEART (in German, HERZ) and HART (in German, HIRSCH) are spelled the way they are spelled. (If it is just to keep the homophones apart could they have been interchanged?) The great difficulty comes with that ubiquitous but chameleon-like digraph EA, which appears in about half of the examples just given. Not being a linguist, I don't profess to understand or explain to a child why the digraph EA in the first example HEART reads /äh/, why in two others (BREAD, well-READ) it reads /e/, why in others (BEAR, PEAR, WEAR[8]) it is pronounced /ä/, in still others (BREAK, GREAT, STEAK) as /ā/, and why, finally, in the rest of them it sounds like /ee/. But this digraph is really an exception. In general, there are some rules to go by. One of the rules (previously mentioned) is that vowel digraphs usually signify long vowel sounds for which there are no equivalent letter symbols. This rule will certainly not hold for BREAD or (well)-READ.[9] According to another rule, the *second* character in a vowel digraph *generally* acts as a kind of retroactive determinant: It makes the first vowel assume its "long" sound, its "name" sound. In compliance with the rule, the AI digraph shown in earlier clusters of word sound as /ā/, the EE sounds as /ee/, and OA, OE or OU as /ō/. But this is a shaky rule at best. It does not hold good for the digraph EI which, e.g., in EIGHT,

HEIGHT, and CON-CEIVE represents three different sounds, with
only the last of them (significantly, a foreign word!) following the rule.
It also does not hold good for IE and OO. But none of the digraphs is
as erratic in indicating a sound as the EA is.

Sometimes we can also blame the mischievous R. One can never
tell what pranks it will play. Often, as in

EAR   DEAR   FEAR   GEAR   HEAR
REAR   YEAR   CLEAR   BEARD

it lets the rule EA = /ee/ prevail, but then in

HEART   HEARTH
PEARL   YEARN   SEARCH
BEAR   PEAR   WEAR

it modifies the EA in three different ways. Its effect on the digraph
AI was discussed earlier. Its effect in this combination is highly de-
pendable: AIR always sounds like ARE, e.g.,

PAIR sounds like PARE (= *pär*)
HAIR sounds like HARE (= *här*)

The role of the R is quite specific. If the last letter in the group
AI-plus-consonant is *any other* consonant but an R, then the sound
value of the digraph is /ā/, not /ä/. The vowel sounds in

PAIR   PAIL   PAIN

are different — one can depend on this — as different as they are in
their respective homophones

PARE   PALE   PANE

One can seldom offer a phonic rule as free of exceptions as this is.
In general, with an R around, one can expect all kinds of difficulties.
Often I can offer only questions, not answers. Why is the /ee/ sound
in VEER spelled EE, whereas in WEIRD it is spelled EI? And why in
SEARCH, BIRCH, and CHURCH is the /ûr/ sound spelled three
different ways? Most examples given earlier suggested that history
and etymology offer an answer and that spelling depends strictly on
word origin. Sometimes, I confess, I am not so sure. SEARCH is cognate with the French CHERCHER; thus to indicate the sound /ûr/
the logical spelling would be SERCH without an A.[10] But why BIRCH

(German, BIRKE) and CHURCH (German, KIRCHE) are spelled two different ways, I cannot tell.

The help phonic rules can offer refers to proper sounding and not to the proper choosing of vowel digraphs; for the latter history and etymology are better guides. An attractive example for this is the word

EIGHT

to which I have referred once before. There I pointed out its Germanic origin as indicated by the silent GH. Here I want to call attention to the fact that in cockneyese and Australese (both archaic ways to pronounce English) the word EIGHT rhymes with RIGHT and HEIGHT.[11] There is a chance that the word originally sounded $\bar{i}t$, before in "good" modern English it became the homophone of ATE, which would explain why it is spelled in such a strange manner. Such assumptions offer keys for quite a few other strangely spelled words.[12] But to offer perhaps an even more reasonable explanation for a number of exceptions, of "irregularly" spelled words, of "irregularly" pronounced digraphs, one must sometimes delve somewhat deeper.

English is also a language with a split personality. While spoken English tends toward greater and greater brevity, greater and greater simplicity in pronunciation (especially in common words in daily usage), written English tends to preserve a visual form: new wine in old bottles. The spoken word

bred

means a thing which is daily prayed for. It is a word in daily usage. Its vowel sound will tend to be short and basic. At the same time, the written form of the word continues to suggest some original word with a double vowel or a long vowel. Perhaps it had a sound like BRE-AD in old English?[13] As far as I can tell, the German, Dutch, and Swedish cognates all carry long vowels.

An even more impressive example of this tendency to shortness and simplicity in spoken basic language is the word

BREAKFAST

It just became too much to state every morning that one will

brāk the *fāhst*

when the word that sounds

brekfest

is so much shorter and so much easier to pronounce. Thus, the pronunciation has changed while the spelling, the "signal image," remained inviolate. That "irregularity of spelling" of everyday words
which so much baffles the foreigner when he begins to study English is often more apparent than real. As this example so vividly
demonstrates, it is often not the spelling which is "irregular": the
spelling follows some old rule or retains the memory of an older pronunciation. It is actually the pronunciation that in a prolonged process of simplification, slowly but surely got "out of order," so that
finally spelling and pronunciation just don't seem to match.

Many other examples could be mustered, among them such
truly basic "everyday" verbs as

(to) LIVE   (to) LOVE   (to) GIVE[14]   (to) COME

all pronounced with a short vowel (and one of them with the original
unchanged Germanic /g/ sound) in spite of the spelling.

One could almost call it a rule that the more common, the
more "everyday," some English word is, the greater the chance that
its spelling and its pronunciation will not fully match. But words like
BREAD and BREAKFAST are still exceptions. Most so-called irregularly spelled words follow, in general, some quite accurately defined
phonic rule or rules. Certain verbs come to mind (they are already
familiar examples), verbs which symbolize some of our most common everyday activities, like

EAT/ATE
SEE/SAW
THINK/THOUGHT

The chances are that such words are monosyllables. And the chances
are that the reader will meet with either modifiers or digraphs (or
both) among their spelling props. The inflection (change of tense)
follows well established rules (an I-related vowel sound turns into
either an /ā/ or /aw/), and the spelling indicates pronunciation accurately. Admittedly, there is *some* unpredictability. Why the first
word, EAT, is spelled with EA, not EE, why SEE (in German SEH-)

and not its homophone SEA (in German, SEE) means the act of vision, only an expert in old German can tell. But as far as phonic problems are concerned, both the present tense forms (EAT, SEE, THINK) and the past tense forms (ATE, SAW, THOUGHT) are defined with the greatest accuracy by rules I have already discussed, by rules of "de-coding", which a student must be taught in the second or third grade!

To my way of thinking there is nothing irregular spellingwise in these three pairs of verb paradigms. On the contrary. The genius of the Germanic languages, their way of expressing a modification in meaning (in this case, a change of tense), manifests itself in this type of verb in the simplest, shortest, most poignant manner, worthy of teacher and student's attention and admiration. Don't alienate the student from this feature by calling it "irregular." There is really no point in aping either the German or the French grammarians who invented the idea of a "strong" or an "irregular" verb inflection. If I were the teacher, I would simply tell students that the past tense of EAT *is* ATE. I am sure they gain nothing by learning that the verb is "strong." Admittedly, and this exactly is my point, if we take any of those long, elaborate Latin- or Greek-derived (non-Germanic!) superstructure, words such as

SUBSTANTI-ATE   ELABOR-ATE   PROCRASTIN-ATE

we can be sure that their inflection is "weak" ("regular"), and that their spelling is predictable. The chances are almost nil that one will find a vowel digraph in them. And if one encounters a modifier, it will be the simplest one, the silent E at the end to make the A in ATE a long vowel. There is no question that the past tense of ELABOR-ATE is ELABOR-AT(E)-ED.

Returning now to the phonic problems posed by vowel digraphs, we must state that in many cases we are, in fact, not dealing with rules, only with "guessing helpers." But guessing is one of the most attractive features of the English spelling procedure. It is the great game of teaching English spelling. It is this game feature which the look-and-say method fails to develop. Words have to be sounded out during this teaching procedure. (No silent reading!) Suddenly a child finds a sounded-out morpheme meaningful. *This* is learning's true reward.

True, our digraph rules are quite shaky, and this we cannot hide
for long. No sooner has the student familiarized himself with the
sound of the digraph OW[15] in words like

ROW   BLOW   CROW
GLOW   TOW   THROW

when we have to teach him that the same digraph represents another
sound value — a diphthong sound — in words like

BROWN   CROWD   CROWN
FOWL   FROWN   HOWL   TOWN

We may want to bring to the student's attention (again some kind of a
phonic rule) the fact that the first alternative more often than not
occupies the end of a word, whereas the latter is found in the middle
of words where it is followed by a consonant. But we will have to add
immediately that this, too, is no law, only a rule, a guessing helper, as
some words have just occurred to us in which the rule does not hold.
Examples in which the rule does not hold (there must be more!) are

BLOWN   THROWN[16]
BROW   HOW   BOW[17]   SOW

And just to complicate matters we shall have to mention once more
that there exists a kind of homophone to the OW digraph, the O-plus-
silent E which, like all silent E's, always occurs at the end of words.
All we can do is to give some examples, like

DOE   FOE   HOE   ROE   TOE

to practice and memorize.

Once the child understands what homophones are and the significance of spelling in identifying them, the teacher can experiment
with a game of word triplets or quadruplets like

HEAR	HERE	HAIR	HARE
MAID	MADE	NEAT	NEED
FEAR	FAIR	FARE	FEEL
PEAR	PAIR	PIER	PEER
HEAL	HEEL	HAIL	HALE
MEAL	MILE	MAIL	MALE
PEAL	PEEL	PAIL	PALE

VEAL	VEIL	VALE	VAIL
MEAT	MEET	MAID	MATE
WHEAL	WHEEL		WHALE
FOOL	FOUL		FOWL
HOLE	WHOLE		HOWL
TOE	TOW	TUNE	TOWN
ROAD	RODE	ROUT	ROOT

In such examples problems are compounded, since not only homophones but also modifiers and digraphs are practiced.

Combinations of this type make teaching lively and add to the challenge one can present to an interested and well-motivated child. Whenever possible we should explain difficulties by history. A child is never too young for this. Children are much cleverer than we think they are. They have to be taken seriously. We don't tell them the story about the stork any more. We talk about chromosomes. Why not tell them how their language has come about? If a child asks why MOVE is not spelled with a digraph, as one might expect, while TOUCH is so spelled, our only possible answer is in terms of history. In spoken language these words became /m/-/oo/-/v/ and /t/-/u/-/ch/ and that's that. But the written tongue retains the memory of the respective Latin and French words in the spelling. English *is* a highbrow language.

A child might also ask why one of those two ubiquitous homophones

TOO   TWO

is spelled the way it is, and why it is the strange letter conglomerate T-W-O which means the number and not T-OO, its regularly spelled sibling. Again the only possible answer is in terms of history. To justify the W in the spelled English word for the spoken *number* /t/-/oo/, I can readily refer, among other examples, to the Czech DVA and the German ZWEI (cognates of the Latin DUO). Both carry a sound that was originally present in Indo-Germanic languages. The sound (the tongue twister) was disposed of in English pronunciation but was retained in the written form. The English *are* traditionalists.

Similar questioning is justified when important but archaic-looking words such as

THOUGH   THROUGH   THOROUGH

are met with, words with a digraph *and* a modifier, pronounced *thō*, *throo*, and *thorō*. Again there is no explanation better than the scientific, the explanation in terms of language history. The teacher might first want to remind the student that in words like

HIGH and THIGH   RIGHT and NIGHT

this silent but modifying GH group has already been met with. She might also want to refer to the respective German word forms

DOCH   DURCH

or to some other cognates in other Germanic tongues, though this might be considered going too far in an elementary teaching situation. She should certainly refer at least in some general way to the fact that English words that contain the letter groups GH or GHT usually[18] are of Germanic (Anglo-Saxon) provenance and originally contained a guttural sound. She should tell the students that this sound was eventually disposed of for the beautification (one might surmise) of the spoken word, while its written traces were retained and were actually turned into a retroactive and almost always silent modifier, a modifier of the letter I in the examples originally given, and of the digraph OU in the examples now considered. Such an explanation will go over quite well in third grade and certainly in fourth.

There is always some logic, some *regula*, behind what an unfortunate (and actually false) attitude presents as "irregularity" or "unnecessary complexity" of English spelling. Here are two words, paradigms of "irregularity," of "unnecessary complexity,"

BROUGHT   THOUGHT

They remind us in their form and structure of the words THOUGH and THOROUGH just discussed, as they, too, each carry the same digraph and the same modifier. They are, of course, the past tenses (and the past participles) of the verb

BRING   THINK

Let us see how "irregular" the declension of these verbs really is.

Let us first of all consider the vowel change. It is anything but irregular. It follows the rule presented earlier:

If the present tense form of a verb contains an E- or I-related sound, a "high" vowel sound (linguists also speak of a "front" vowel

sound), then in the past tense the vowel is bound to change to an A, O, or U (a "low" or "back" vowel sound).[19]

We noted at that time that the same rule is being followed by German verbs. Thus, we find that the present tense of the cognate German words is

BRING(E)   DENK(E)

changing to

BRACHTE   DACHTE

in the past tense. German grammarians will categorize these verbs as subject to a "strong" declension. The respective endings of our two paradigm English verb roots in the present tense are -ING and -INK, those of their German cognates are -ING and -ENK. In the past tense both English verbs end in a -T, and the German verbs in -TE. This type of ending is rather regular for both languages. In fact, in German the past tense of all so-called "weak" verbs (considered to be the more regular ones) ends in -TE while in English the past tense of all so-called "regular" verbs ends in -ED. The -T ending (a linguistic relative of the D sound) in English verbs is a kind of compromise solution, quite often encountered, neither "weak" nor "strong." Again all this follows rules and brings us finally into the domain of still another rule, a rule we have repeatedly invoked, a rule that tells us that the Germanic letter conglomerate CH or GH (for the guttural sound /kh/) changes into a retroactive, silent vowel modifier in the cognate English words.[20] Thus, we have

English BROUGHT (= *brawt*)   German BRACH-TE (= *brakhte)*
English THOUGHT (= *thawt*)   German DACH-TE (= *dakhte)*

the GH modifying the sound of the digraph OU. There is, in fact, nothing in these "irregularly" spelled, "difficult," "unnecessarily complex" words

BROUGHT   THOUGHT

that could not be covered down to the minutest detail by some rule.[21]

A few paragraphs earlier I used the expression: "The English are traditionalists." I also used the expression "English is a highbrow language." Once I referred to its "split personality." What I have tried time and again was to show how English spelled words endeavored to retain some of their original form elements (elements usually recognizable in Germanic cognates or traceable to roots in Latin) in spite of all the changes in pronunciation brought about by time (and I mean centuries). Indeed, if one is in the wrong mood one would almost be inclined to call this a kind of schizophrenia of the English tongue: Spelling more often than not remains historical, rigid, and unchangeable, while pronunciation changes freely, haphazardly, it often seems, but, in fact, it follows certain well-established laws of phonetic drift.[22]

The word, TWO, discussed earlier, is a good example of these antagonistic tendencies. The letter W was retained in the spelled word but eliminated as a tongue twister from the pronounced one (in English, not in Czech or German). Another pertinent example is

SWORD (German, SCHWERT)

for the same phenomenon.

At this juncture, I might refer to some other earlier given example pairs,

WRITE and WRIGHT   KNIGHT and KNAVE

to demonstrate the difference in approach (I might almost say, the difference in spirit) of German and English, a difference that is striking in view of the fact that both are Germanic tongues. In each of these English words a crowding initial consonant, once present, has been dropped from pronunciation, but retained in the spelling. The Germans, too, dropped the sound of the initial W in REISSEN and RICHTEN, cognate words to the first two examples. But they also dropped the letter from their spelling. On the other hand, they retained the initial K in the last two examples, KNECHT and KNABE, both in their pronunciation *and* in their spelling. No schizophrenia. (I am not making a value judgment. I am merely relating a fact.)

But there are no generally valid statements in linguistics. More often than not, English and German solved linguistics problems quite similarly. A good example is an arrangement sometimes used in English to indicate the plural of some rather common nouns, an arrangement that often has the meaningless adjective "irregular" attached

to it. Some examples have already been given, but I may as well repeat them (with one or two added):

LOUSE/LICE   MOUSE/MICE   (HOUSE/HOUSES!)

FOOT/FEET   GOOSE/GEESE

All these words are Germanic, and their cognate German plurals
are earmarked by what linguists call an *umlaut,* that is, by a shift in
base vowel from "back" to "front." (Germans usually call it from
"low" to "high.") Thus, we find in German:

LAUS/LÄUSE   MAUS/MÄUSE   HAUS/HÄUSER

FUSS/FÜSSE   GANS/GÄNSE

This impressively simple, unequivocal spelling arrangement was not,
as such, adopted in written English. The "umlaut" concept is foreign
to •English.[23] Still, a change in vowel sound was taken over into
spoken English, and it had to be indicated in some manner. There
was certainly no simpler and more economic way to indicate this
shift than by the use of a silent E (-ICE) or of a digraph (EE), the
phonetic values of which are unequivocally given and very similar to
the phonetic values in the respective German cognates. LOUSE/-
LICE and LAUS/LÄUSE sound very similar, and so do FOOT/-
FEET, and FUSS/FÜSSE.

By the way, the choice of the simpler digraph EE also separates
the word FEET from a homophone,

FEAT

which gives me opportunity once more to reiterate, with love, that
English spelling is never haphazard, seldom irregular, and historically almost always justified and justifiable. Analyzing the homophones

FEET   FEAT

it will be clear that it is the second of the two variants which (through
the French word FAIT) finally came down from the Latin FACTUM.
Hence the letter A in the spelling. FEET, on the other hand, is the
cognate of the German FÜSSE. (In vulgar German and in Yiddish
the plural of FÜSSE almost sounds like *fees.*) One can be sure that it
is the spelled word FEET, with the simpler digraph, that signifies a

part of our anatomy — not FEAT, the word with that sophisticated digraph EA in its spelled form.

There are some further obvious questions a child might ask: Why are there only five vowels in the English alphabet when there are at least twenty vowel sounds in the spoken language? Why, on the other hand, is there such a conspicuous superabundance of letters that signify the sound /k/? Again the answer can only be given in terms of history. English spelling, we must repeat, is conservative, and since in the Latin alphabet, which is used to write English, there were only five vowels, that is where things began and ended. All vowel sounds other than the five basic vowel sounds must therefore be symbolized by modifiers or digraphs, with a modicum of guessing added to make it a challenge.

The letter Y, a kind of sixth vowel, is traceable to the Greeks. Its inclusion adds some welcome variety to the English alphabet, so poor in vowel symbols. It is half vowel, half consonant, and it is important that the teacher explain the difference between the "consonant" Y in

YEARN   YIELD   YOKE   (JOKE!)
BOY   TOY   (BUY!)
LAW-YER   SAW-YER

and the "vowel" Y, which can be short, as in

LOVELY   EASY

or long, as in

BY   DRY

The short-vowel Y has always seemed to me just a kind of embellishment on I, without any influence on pronunciation: Y = I = /i/. The long-vowel Y deserves some further consideration in a chapter on phonics. Here are two clusters of words ending in a vowel Y:

BY DRY FLY FRY PLY TRY SHY WHY
RAY BRAY LAY CLAY PLAY TRAY

The teacher might explain that the Y is simply an indicator of a long-sounding I (= /ī/), in the examples of the first row while in the examples of the second row AY is just a variant of the digraph AI (=/ā/), again embellished at end of the word.

But why, a bright child will ask, is the Y pronounced /i/ at the end of a great many other words, as it is in

LOVELY   EASY

the words mentioned a paragraph or so earlier? There must be some rule to follow!

The best a teacher can do under such circumstances is to interpolate some notions about the accent in words and about syllables that modify the meaning of other syllables. Take the examples given in the first cluster:

BY   DRY   FLY   etc.

The teacher should not fail to point out that these words are all monosyllables, with Y being the only vowel. The accent or stress is necessarily on this syllable. Moreover, they are "open" syllables (they end in a vowel), and stressed open syllables "prefer" long vowel sounds. Thus, the chances are that the Y will sound like /ī/. In contradistinction, in the following selection of words with the Y ending,

EASY   EERY   TAWDRY (adjectives)
BERRY   FERRY (nouns)
BURY   CARRY   TARRY   WORRY (verbs)

we face a different situation. There are two syllables to every one of these words (some adjectives, some nouns, some verbs), with the accent on the first, the actual "meaning giving" syllable. The second syllable is unstressed (of secondary significance) and unstressed syllables (even if "open") tend to carry short vowel sounds. Thus, the chances are that the Y sounds /i/. Once more a kind of "rule" is born. And once more clusters of words can be presented to instill this rule into the student's mind.

But there is even more to be learned from words in another cluster of examples:

BARE-LY   CLEAR-LY   FREE-LY
GREAT-LY   MAIN-LY   SLY-LY   TRU(E)-LY

The first syllable in these words is the sole "meaning carrier," while the syllable LY that ends the words is merely a "meaning modifier." It is nothing but a grammatical device to turn adjectives like

BARE   CLEAR   FREE

into adverbs. The morphemes BARE, CLEAR, FREE, etc., carry, so to speak, the burden of meaning. The ending LY only modifies, adjusts these words, to fit them, if necessary, into appropriate sentence structures. We can say:

a man is FREE

We can also say:

a man breathes FREELY

and we will never doubt that LY in the latter sentence has not changed the meaning of the word, merely adjusted it. The syllable will be unstressed; its vowel component is bound to sound short.

There is no harm if the teacher brings to the student's attention in this connection that there are other kinds of meaning modifiers which can be attached to meaning-giving (one can also call them "meaning-carrying") "roots." In the last cluster of examples, the "meaning-giving" syllable was *followed* by the meaning modifier; in others it can be preceded by one. In the first case we speak of a "suffix," in the latter of a "prefix." Then there are words with both a prefix and a suffix to modify the word's basic meaning. Neither of these syllables, the teacher might add, is normally stressed. Neither of these syllables ordinarily carries a long vowel.

There is no reason why "long" words, derived words, should be avoided even at an elementary level of instruction. For the student taught by the "code" method, such words offer no difficulties. Generally it is only the meaning-giving syllable (the syllable that carries the stress) whose spelling and pronunciation have to be watched, and which offer phonic intricacies.[24] But the suffixes and prefixes offer no phonic problems, no pronunciation problems.

With this new rule (if one can call it a rule), many new words can be presented and the child's reading vocabulary increased tremendously. The teacher will do best if at this point she introduces clusters of words with prefixes, with each cluster demonstrating one particular prefix, such as

A-BIDE A-FLOAT A-FOOT A-FRAID A-GAPE A-GLOW
A-LONE A-LOOF A-NEW A-STIR (A-GENT!)

BE-COME BE-GET BE-HEAD BE-LIE
BE-STIR BE-STOW BE-QUEATH[25]

Then the teacher should present words with both a prefix and a suffix, words of three syllables, with the middle syllable meaning-giving and stressed, and a meaning modifier on each end, e.g.,

A-BID(E)-ING BE-COM(E)-ING
BE-LOV(E)-ED BE-NIGHT-ED

The last word is an especially attractive example of the ease with which the reading of compounded words can be mastered, and demonstrates the advantages of our phonic-analytic technique in any attack on "long" words. Once the student has learned to "handle" the word NIGHT, the longer word offers no new obstacles. For the poor child taught according to the look-and-say technique,

NIGHT   BENIGHTED

would be two words to be memorized by repetition. For a child trained by phonics there is nothing new to be learned.

But let me finish my discussion of the letter Y. There is, in fact, little to add. It will do no harm if older students are told about the rather common occurrence of the letter Y in words of Greek origin. A simple but excellent example is

TYPE (noun or verb)

The word is a monosyllable; thus, it carries a stress in the very nature of things. In English it is pronounced with a long $/\bar{\text{i}}/$ sound whatever the pronunciation of the root word was in Greek. (It certainly did not sound $/\bar{\text{i}}/$.)

When one looks for other words of Greek origin that contain a Y, one will find that quite a number of "learned" words begin, for example, with the prefix SYN- (SYL- or SYM-), and that they all have something to do with "together." Since the syllable is a prefix, a meaning modifier, the chances are that it will be pronounced with a short /i/.

The meaning of the following examples

SYNAGOGUE   SYNOD   SYNTAX   SYNONYM   SYLLABLE
SYMBOL   SYMPHONY[26]   SYMPOSIUM(!)
SYNDICATED   SYNOPTIC(!)

is generally known to the more advanced student, and if not, it does
not matter; one has to be able to read words the meaning of which he
does not yet know. That is how one "learns."

It should be noted, by the way (for future reference), that in this
particular cluster of examples it is the prefix with the short /i/ sound
which (with one or two exceptions) carries the accent. Thus, it is not
always the root word upon which the stress falls.

It might be interesting to point out that it is the conservative Anglo-Saxon who
will stick to the "correct" spelling. We call it

SYMPHONY

the carefree Italian brazenly spells the word as

SINFONIA

Since the child with a reading problem (certainly his parents!)
will quite likely meet with that ominous word

DYS-LEXIA

there is no harm in mentioning that DYS- is also a meaning modifier
of Greek origin and simply indicates that something is wrong. (It's
the reading in this instance.)

One more item: There is a Y in one of the homophones

LIE and LYE   DIE and DYE

for which my usual explanation (or excuse) is separation of homophones. But why

RYE

is spelled the way it is, I don't know.

As far as the three consonants C,[27] K, Q are concerned (three
consonants that today, to our ear, sound the same), the teacher must
again remind the questioning child of the conservatism of English
spelling and also of the Latin (and, indirectly, Greek) origin of the

English alphabet. How C and Q came to English from Latin and K to English through the Greek alphabet is an interesting story to which intelligent children will listen eagerly. Of course, the teacher must know about this story to be able to tell it. Unfortunately, many teachers of reading at the elementary level have never been exposed to a study of the origins of the English language, let alone a study of the history of the English alphabet. It is no wonder that sometimes they themselves don't know how to spell some words. How can they teach spelling except by rote, by the look-and-learn method? In any event, the chances are today that words starting with C are of Latin (or Greek) origin:

CAMP   CANCEL   COMFORT   CONFLICT
CURE   CATALOG   (CAR!)

while words starting with K,

KEEP   KIN   KING   KNOWLEDGE

are not. (But this is not a hard and fast rule.)

The Q has a rather limited role in today's English. It figures only as the first half of the consonant complex Qu = /kv/ in both Anglo-Saxon words such as

QUEEN

and Latin words such as

QUARTER   QUASI

In some words (adapted through French),

ANTIQUE   TECHNIQUE,

the spelling remanded while the second sound was lost. The answer to the questioning child is then that the Latin, Greek, or Anglo-Saxon words just carried their C or K or Q with them. It must be impressed upon the child that *nothing in this is haphazard* or willfully chosen. The heart of the child who learns to read English should be imbued with love and respect for the English language. Granted, sometimes spelling could have been simpler. Granted, sometimes the difficulties are frustrating. But certainly, English spelling represents an heroic course steered between the Scylla of pronunciation and the

Charybdis of tradition. English spelling is meaningful and purposeful. Why otherwise all the effort?

Of course, one cannot help getting exasperated sometimes. Why does the word

LEAGUE

need a digraph, a modifier, and a demodifier to stand for three simple phonemes

/l/-/ee/-/g/

This *is* much too complicated.[28] And there are other words altogether without logic. Why are WOMAN and WOMEN spelled with an O? Why is the morpheme *shoogar* spelled SUGAR? Why is SHOE (in German, SCHUH, though in Dutch SCHOE) written as it is and pronounced as it is when (a) the old /oo/ sound of both the German and the Dutch has been retained and (b) the digraph OE, as in TOE, is usually pronounced /ō/? Why, indeed, is the word not spelled SHOO? Similar problems present themselves with WHO and TO (in German, ZU). Both are much too important and ubiquitous words. Some irregularity is almost to be expected. Probably the shorter their spelled form, the better. One just has to learn how they are spelled, in the look-and-say manner, without asking questions.

Of course, I try my best to find explanations and though I don't have enough background knowledge to be sure that my explanations are "scientifically" correct, at least they represent an attitude. I do provide reasons, which is better than referring to spelling "irregularities."

The other day a boy asked why

PEOPLE

is spelled the way it is. "Isn't this highly irregular?"
I told the boy that the word comes from the Latin

POPULUS

and thus the spelled English word should contain an O. I also reminded the boy of the "rule" of vowel digraphs; they usually indicate that the first of the two vowels should be pronounced in its "long" form. And, finally, I reiterated the "rule" that pronunciation has precedence. We pronounce the word as

/p/-/ee/-/p/-/l/

so the first vowel should be an E (the "long" pronunciation of which is /ee/). And since we do need a digraph and have the tradition of the Latin POPULUS, the letter O is a rather logical though somewhat outlandish choice for the digraph's second vowel. I don't know how much merit these types of explanations have. But my discussion made the hour lively, and I am sure this boy will never forget that the morpheme *peepl* is spelled PEOPLE and will not worry about "irregularity."

As for the separation of homophones by differential spelling, I confess I sometimes wonder if it is really worth the trouble. Hungarian, too, has a number of homophones, but since spelling in that language is phonetic, Hungarian homophones are always homographs at the same time.

The English language has some homographs (I am not aware of many).[29] Some sound differently, depending on meaning:

(to) BOW	BOW (and arrow)
(the) WIND	(to) WIND
(a) TEAR (liquid)	(to) TEAR (something)
(to) LEAD	LEAD (metal)

Some are also homophones:

(to) MAIL	MAIL (armor)	
SEAL (animal)	SEAL (verb)	
STEER	(to) STEER	
EAR	EAR (corn)	
(a) BEAR	(to) BEAR	
(a) LOAF	(to) LOAF	
SOLE (fish)	SOLE (foot)	SOLE (alone)

I don't think that this could ever cause any confusion. Syntax and the arrangement of words within phrases readily take care of meaning in English as well as in Hungarian.

In cases like these, where questions arise for which answers are not readily forthcoming, the wisdom of the teacher means much. Sometimes illogical things have to be accepted simply by consent (like the name of the month of November). The growing up of a child can be measured by the child's acceptance of things that are meaningful or advantageous for communication; they don't *always* have to be true or logical. As my mother used to say: Only children and morons *always* tell the truth.

NOTES

[1]The difference can be illustrated by the difference between the vowel sounds in the English words HAT and BED. They are not interchangeable. Hungarian orthography failed to create different symbols for these two quite different sounds.

[2]I will, of course, repeatedly ask: "Do you know this word?" "Do you know what the word means?" After all, one helps build a vocabulary whenever one can. But all this is incidental. The emphasis is on "de-coding."

[3]The explanation offered in connection with such words as LIE or PIE is a matter of choice. One can say that they are simply examples of the silent E lengthening the sound of the preceding vowel I. But one can also say that they are instances in which the diagraph IE is pronounced /ī/.

[4]This again is a matter of attitude. One can list OE and OW as digraphs with a long /ō/ sound value. But one can also list them as examples of the silent E and the modifying W respectively. As for the letter combination OE, to list it as an example of the silent E might even be the more correct classification seeing that it occurs only at the end of words.

[5]OU and AU are often encountered as digraphs in connection with the retroactive vowel modifier GH or GHT, as in BOUGH *(bou)* or BOUGHT *(bawt)*.

[6]I confess I do not know why in the first cluster the /ee/ is spelled EE, why in the second it is spelled IE. I also don't know why the same /ee/ sound sometimes associates with a diagraph EI, as in

         CON-CEIVE   RE-CEIVE   CEILING   RE-CEIPT   SEIZE

Perhaps it has something to do with the period during which French words like RECEIVRE (in modern French, RECEVOIR) found their entry into the English thesaurus of words. (The explanation would not hold for CEILING coming, as it seems, from the French CIEL.)

[7]The sound of the digraph OO (=/oo/) can be short (=/ŏŏ/), as in FOOT or long (= /o͞o/) as in ROOM. I don't think that this will cause any difficulties in teaching. I plan to neglect the difference. The child will know most of these words by sound (they are in his spoken vocabulary) and will automatically add the proper length value to *foot* or *room*.

[8]In this one instance (all three examples end in R!) one suspects the overriding modifying effect of the R.

[9]Other examples in which EA sounds /e/ are HEAD, SPREAD, TREAD, THREAD, WEALTH. There are, I am sure, many more, too many to call exceptions. (I agree with the "meaning" school that such words must be memorized. It is impossible to give the history of the spelling of each of such words to pupils in grade school).

[10]The only mitigating circumstance is that in CHERCHER the vowel sound is short while the digraph in SEARCH a long vowel is indicated. To this, one could, of course, object that in SERVE, etc. (cf. p. 45), the vowel sound is also long and still orthography indicates no digraph. To answer this objection one must refer to the historical structuring of the English language, about which more will be said in the chapters that follow. The English felt free to assimilate French words into their peculiar spelling system while Latin words were sacrosanct! The French CHERCHER could be twisted to the fancies of English spelling, but the Latin SERVARE is inviolate.

[11]In modern German EI sounds like /ī/ as REICH or WEIN.

[12]If it has not already been done (which is unlikely), it would make a worthwhile Ph.D. thesis for someone to analyze strangely spelled English words from this particular point of view.

[13]Note the pronunciation *bre-yud* in parts of the Southern United States.

[14]It might have some significance, it certainly is worth noting, that another truly "basic" verb,

GET

has also retained the old sound.

[15]I have in an earlier part of this volume referred to the combination O-plus-W as vowel plus retroactive modifier. Here I refer to it as digraph. Both concepts serve as aids to teaching and are not contradictory.

[16]These two words are not real exceptions. They are so-called past participles, derived, respectively, from BLOW and THROW.

[17]This word can actually be pronounced both ways and has different meanings when it is pronounced one or the other way.

[18]The word "usually" just had to be added, though I could also have said "in the overwhelming majority." Offhand I can mention no more than three or four verbs whose past tense carries a digraph and ends in GHT and which have no German cognates known to me. They are:

BUY/BOUGHT
TEACH/TAUGHT
CATCH/CAUGHT
DISTRACT/DISTRAUGHT

Still, at least the first two are (according to Webster) of Germanic (old Anglo-Saxon or Gothic) origin, and only the last one patently comes from the Latin. This, then, would be a true exception. (I guess it is a mistake perpetuated.) How to explain the strange digraph in the word BUY (pronounced $b\bar{\imath}$) remains a problem. This finally brings us to words such as:

COUGH   ROUGH   TOUGH
TROUGH   ENOUGH   (BOUGH!   DOUGH!)

and

LAUGH   DRAUGHT   (DROUGHT!)

all Germanic words with the relatively rare digraph OU and the even rarer digraph AU. The original guttural sound (indicated by the letter group GH) in these examples was not disposed of (is not silent) but is pronounced /f/. They are best memorized as phonic peculiarities.

[19]I use the highly unorthodox term *anti-umlaut* to describe this rule.

[20] We had several examples of this earlier, outstanding among them being

English RIGHT (= $r\bar{\imath}t$)   German RECHT (= *rekht*)

the GH modifying the sound of the letter I into /ī/.

[21]As one looks back at his linguistic prejudices, one finds less and less of what is haphazard, more and more of a prevalence of "rules." Somewhere earlier I said that auxiliary verbs are so common and so ubiquitous that one need not even bother to find anything in their different forms to suggest some rule. I must have been wrong. I note the two verb forms:

(he) HAS   (he) HAD

One can bet any amount of money that it is the word ending in D that signifies the past tense and not the other one. Even that most "irregular" auxiliary verb

(to) BE

follows some rules; in the past participle form it turns into

BEEN

a form whose N ending is also the ending found in the past participle of other verbs, such as

SEE   SEEN
DRAW   DRAWN
SHOW   SHOWN

and so on. The same holds true for another very irregular verb,

DO   DOES   DID   DONE

The form for the past tense ends in D and for the past participle in NE. Rules break through everywhere; the inflections are as "regular" as possible. What is irregular is the pronunciation. To give some random examples:

HAVE   ARE   DOES   DONE

do not follow the established pronunciation rules (the A in HAVE is short, etc.). But even this follows a "rule": vowels tend to become short in words often used. (Think of the example BREAKFAST, discussed earlier.)

[22]It will be worth noting that even the "schizophrenia" of English pronunciation and spelling is limited to vowels. We don't mind leaving the O in MOVE unchanged and pronounce it /oo/; we retain the historical spelling although pronunciation has changed. But there is no such adjustability when the pronunciation requires a /z/ as in APPEASE; we don't spell it APPEACE.

[23]In fact, it is only the concept that is foreign. In reality English, too, avails itself of it. In the examples we have just discussed, there is a shift of vowel from "back" to "front" (this, and not the two dots on the A or O or U, is the essence of the "umlaut"). Note that we are dealing with nouns and that the change is from singular to plural. Let us then call a "quasi-umlaut" what in

LOUSE/LICE changes OU (= /ou/) to I (= /ī/)

and in

FOOT/FEET changes OO (= /oo/) to EE (= /ee/)

Somewhere in our previous discussion we gave a whole cluster of examples of what we might call a kind of "anti-umlaut," a change from "front" to "back" root vowel. Note that these words were all verbs and the change has been from present to past tense. The English examples for this "anti-umlaut" were

FIGHT   FOUGHT
WRITE   WROTE

The German examples showing a similar trend, were

SING(E)   SANG
BRING(E)   BRACHTE

and so on (cf. p. 45). It all follows strict rules. Nothing haphazard. All one has to adopt is the principle of "umlaut" for nouns, of "anti-umlaut" for verbs. Everything then falls into its proper place, and we don't have to bother calling LICE an irregular plural for LOUSE. Even the fact that we spell the word LICE and not LISE is economical and significant: The pronunciation of ICE is constant, but the pronunciation of ISE is variable; an S may sound /s/ or /z/, but a C before an E can only be pronounced /s/.

[24]The examples were actually so chosen as to emphasize the difficulties. Every one of them is a "problem." In BARE there are two retroactive modifiers, in CLEAR and GREAT the same vowel digraph is pronounced in two different ways, etc.

[25]In the last example (BEQUEATH) I have purposely chosen a word that 99% of the regular readers of the *New York Daily News* will never encounter in their reading, a word which a third or fourth grader will find he cannot understand. I am sure it never occurs in any look-and-say text. It is a rarely used and difficult word. But all this does no matter. If the reader is ever confronted with the word, he should not have a problem with "de-coding." That is all a phonics technique of teaching reading must and will guarantee.

[26]The Y at the end is again just an embellishment. The Romans wrote SYMPHONIA; the English discarded the vowel A and made a Y out of the I.

[27]As already noted, C before E and I sounds not like /k/ but like /s/. Why the sound /s/ is spelled as C in some words and as S in others is purely a problem in etymology. The example

CERTAIN versus SERVE

was given earlier.

[28]As I reread this statement, I find that my judgment was much too rash. The complexity has good historic reasons. Reading the word aloud, I find that it sounds exactly the same way as the French word

LIGUE

from which (though the original root is Latin) it actually derives. As happened with so many French (more accurately, Latin-French) imports, the root word became "incorporated," so to speak, into the English spelling system. (More about that in the next chapter.) Had the codifiers of English spelling taken the word over unchanged, the English reader would have been wont to read

$$\overline{\text{lig}}$$

looking at the silent E at the end of the word with English (not French) eyes. He will not now do this since the vowel digraph EA with the preferred sound /ee/ was substituted for the I. I find the same solution in a related word, COL-LEAGUE (French, COL-LÈGUE, from Latin, COL-LEGA) with the right pronunciation duly indicated within the English spelling system. (The French ending GUE was left untouched in both examples and indicates that the end consonant is to be pronounced and should sound /g/, not /j/. (The French COL-LÈGE and the English COL-LEGE, carry no demodifier and are pronounced accordingly.)

[29]There exists a group of Latin-origin compounded words, each of which has two slightly different meanings for one spelled form. A word like

ELABOR-ĀTE

is a homograph of sorts: it can be a verb, in which case the last syllable sounds *at;* it can also be an adjective, in which case the last syllable is pronounced *et.*

CHAPTER FIVE

*The Three-Layered Structure of the English Language:
The Basic (Anglo-Saxon) Vocabulary — The "Assimi-
lated" Latin-French Contribution — The Latin-Greek
Superstructure — More About the Accent in Half-Long and
Long English Words: Rules and Logic in the Placement of
Stress — Meaning Modifiers: "Meaningful" Meaning
Modifiers vs. "Simple" Meaning Modifiers*

As the reader will have noticed, up to now I have tried to restrict my
discussion of phonics to monosyllabic words. They are the backbone
of the English language. Practically all rules of phonics, of spelling
and pronunciation, of modifiers, and of digraphs can be mastered by
working on monosyllables, on "short" words that are well within a
child's vocabulary, on the vocabulary upon which, as I have already
remarked, all our teaching of reading is based, whatever the technique or philosophy to which we confess. They are — the term is
justified — "basic" words. Dissyllables, "half-long" words, and especially polysyllables, "long" words, are words the child generally
learns later in life, though the radio and television have brought many
of them into the simplest home. The majority of "short" words are
Anglo-Saxon or even earlier words. "Half-long" and "long" words
generally come from Latin or Greek (the "half-long" words usually
through French) to signify more conceptual, less concrete acts, qualities, or things. Here are some examples. First, some short verbs:

EAT DRINK SLEEP WORK LIVE PLAY
SPEAK FIGHT FEEL CRY SEE HEAR
THINK ACT(!) GIVE TAKE HOLD

85

They are all monosyllables.[1] So are the adjectives

GOOD BAD LONG SHORT TALL STRAIGHT
HARD SOFT WARM COLD SWEET BITTER(!)

and so are also the nouns:

BIRTH LIFE DEATH LOVE PAIN(!) HEAD
HAND HEART FRIEND GOD MAN[2]

They are all "basic" words. In contrast, here are some "half-long"
words:

AB-DUCT AD-MIRE COM-MIT CON-FIRM DE-CEIVE
DI-VIDE E-RECT EX-PRESS IN-CITE PER-FORM
PRE-PARE PRO-CEED RE-FUSE SUR-PRISE TRANS-LATE

(all of them happen to be verbs), and some "long" words (syllabized
for easy reading):

AD-MIR-ABLE   IN-CINER-A-TOR
PRO-GRESS-IVE   CO-OR-DIN-A-TION
IN-TOLER-ANT   PER-MISS-ION
E-STAB-LISH-MENT   GYM-NA-SI-UM(!)
CO-RON-A-TION(!)   TE-LE-VI-SION(!)

(some of them adjectives, some of them nouns). They certainly are
not "basic." Nor are they Anglo-Saxon in origin.[3]

Let us first direct our attention to the cluster of "half-long"
words! A student of some maturity can easily be made to realize that
(1) the first syllable of this type of word is generally a so-called prefix,
a meaning-modifying starter syllable with some definite connotation[4]
which he can easily learn (there are only a handful of them) and that
(2) what follows, the root word,[5] is subject to the same kind of spelling analysis as the monosyllables with which he has already become
familiar. As far as "long" words are concerned, chances are that
here, too, the first syllable is a prefix (the exceptions in the
last cluster of words are marked by "!"), that what follows is usually
a Latin root, and that what then follows is another "affix," a so-called
suffix. Structured in this manner, "half-long" words and "long"
words generally are concept words and only occasionally the names
of overt acts or qualities or of "real" things. As far as the spelling of
"long" words is concerned, the student will note, to his pleasant sur-

prise, that it is actually much more consistent than that of many a "short" word and even "half-long" word, that there are hardly any exceptions or irregularities to worry about, and especially that difficult vowel digraphs are hardly ever encountered.

Preparing a child to master more-than-one-syllable words, I usually jot down the second syllable, the root syllable of two-syllable "half-long" words, like the ones I have just clustered haphazardly (chances are that they are of Latin origin) and then add some familiar, "basic" (chances are, Anglo-Saxon), one-syllable word, whenever I find one, for a comparison of their phonic problems:

(AB)	-	DUCT	
(AD)	-	MIRE	FIRE
(COM)	-	MIT	HIT
(CON)	-	FIRM	FIR
(DE)	-	CEIVE	SIEVE
(DI)	-	VIDE	WIDE
(E)	-	RECT	
(EX)	-	PRESS	DRESS
(IN)	-	CITE	BITE
(PER)	-	FORM	
(PRE)	-	PARE	HARE
(PRO)	-	CEED	DEED
(RE)	-	FUSE	USE[6]
(SUR)	-	PRISE	PRIZE
(TRANS)	-	LATE	GATE

It is one of the pleasantly peculiar quirks of the English tongue that it has managed to cover a great many originally Latin words with English garb. This can be demonstrated with some of the last given examples: The Latin roots,

DUCere	MIRAri	MITTere
CITAre	PARAre	CEDere

have in the end become thoroughly Anglicized in both spelling and pronunciation. As far as phonic problems are concerned, they are as English as the Anglo-Saxon words I have used for comparison. I have repeatedly referred to the English as traditionalists who would not think of changing as much as the Y in SYMPHONY or dropping a W from WRITE. With this new observation I am not contradicting that view. English is at one and the same time traditionalistic and boldly utilitarian. It is this miraculous multifacetedness that makes English that supreme tool of communication which it is.

Let us once more return to those half-long words, generally Latin words, which came into English through French, the cluster

AB-DUCT   AD-MIRE   etc.

tabulated earlier.

As the two juxtaposed columns of words show, the spelling and pronunciation rules are the same for the short Anglo-Saxon words and the roots of the half-long French-Latin words. These words form the second structural level of English. Many are "concept" words but they are not yet "learned" words. They are words quasi-"assimilated," quasi-"incorporated" into today's conceptualized[7] basic English. In contradistinction, the really long words (the "learned" words, the new words) follow the original Greek or Latin purely phonetic spelling. *They are the words that offer no phonic problems.* Thus, in the long run the spelling of long words, of Greco-Roman superstructure words, is in fact simpler and easier than that of the basic words, the Anglo-Saxon words. What weighs so heavily in the spelling of English words (the Anglo-Saxon words and the "assimilated" Latin-French words) is homophony and digraph vowels, to which I have devoted ample time. None of these applies to the vast *thesaurus* of superstructure words in which spelling and pronunciation are almost[8] as unequivocal as, say, in Hungarian. It should indeed be evident that long words such as

TE-LE-VI-SION   CO-OR-DIN-A-TION   E-STAB-LISH-MENT

are much easier to read and pronounce (when divided into syllables) than the Anglo-Saxon monosyllables

HEAD   HEART   GRANGE   STRENGTH

words most difficult to master either in dictation or on sight. All that students have to learn (once and for all) is the strange pronunciation of some endings, like -SION, -TION, -OUS, -TIOUS, and the placement of the accent. Placing the accent is, in fact, a problem inseparable from the phonics of words of more than one syllable.

Some guidelines offered themselves rather readily, and I have already suggested them:

1. Simple two-syllable words very often consist of a "basic" monosyllable and an affix.

2. Whether the affix, the added syllable, is a prefix or a suffix, the accent falls naturally and preferentially on the meaning-giving syllable, the root word.

3. Prefixes or suffixes are generally unstressed, and their vowel will almost always be found to be a short one.

The clusters

RARE-LY	CLEAR-LY	FREE-LY etc.
A-BIDE	A-FLOAT	A-FOOT etc.
BE-COME	BE-GET	BE-HEAD etc.

(see p. 73), all basic words (most of them Anglo-Saxon words) with a meaning modifier added, offered a goodly number of examples for the validity of these rules.

The same rules seem to hold for the two-syllable words given in the cluster

AB-DUCT   AD-MIRE   COM-MIT   etc.

French or Latin, the roots of which, have been quasi-assimilated into the "basic" English language with all its phonic problems. However, to other words, some also two-syllable words, words which remained part of the nonincorporated superstructure (let us not be afraid to call them foreign words), these rules cannot be applied with any assurance.[9] In fact, in the case of some "learned," "unassimilated" words with the prefix SYN-, we found that the accent fell on the prefix. (See p. 75.) With considerable uneasiness, I left the impression at the time that this might be just an unpleasant exception. But that, patently, is not the case since other similar examples can be quoted — Greek words with a variety of prefixes:

ANA-GRAM		
CATA-LOG		
DIA-GRAM	DIA-LOG	DIA-PHRAGM,
EPI-GRAM	EPI-LOG	EPI-SODE
META-PHOR		
PRO-GRAM	PRO-LOG	
PROTO-COL, etc.		

Let us once more look at the clusters of words to which we have, with such assurance, applied what seemed to be some reasonable rules. In the example clusters

A-BIDE   A-FLOAT   etc.
BE-COME BE-GET   etc.

(which were root words with a prefix), in the cluster

BARE-LY   CLEAR-LY   etc.

(which were root words with a suffix), and in

A-BID(E)-ING   BE-COM(E)-ING   etc.,

(with a prefix and a suffix), the prefixes and suffixes were truly and merely meaning modifiers. They left the basic meaning of the root words unchanged. This is not so in the examples which started with the prefixes SYN-, ANA-, DIA-, etc. In all these instances we have been dealing with meaning-modifying prefixes which *themselves have meaning.* All we have to do is to rearrange our clusters

ANA-LOG   CATA-LOG   DIA-LOG   EPI-LOG
ANA-GRAM DIA-GRAM EPI-GRAM PRO-GRAM etc.[10]

to demonstrate this significant difference.

Perhaps it is here that the difference finds its explanation. Perhaps it is their being meaningful meaning modifiers that makes certain prefixes worthy, so to speak, to carry the accent? But here again we would arrive at a false conclusion. All we have to do is to take a second look at the original cluster of Latin-French verbs

AB-DUCT   AD-MIRE   etc.

to discover that they too carry meaningful meaning modifiers. It will be best to rearrange the cluster of examples (and make some appropriate additions) to show that a change of these prefixes also changes meaning while, of course, the constancy of the root word assures a certain constancy of the meaning at the same time. Here are some examples:

AB-DUCT	IN-DUCE	PRO-GRESS(!)	AD-MIT
CON-DUCT	PRO-DUCE(!)	RE-GRESS	COM-MIT
DE-DUCT	RE-DUCE	TRANS-GRESS	RE-MIT
IN-DUCT	SE-DUCE		SUB-MIT
PRO-DUCT(!)			TRANS-MIT

COM-POSE	DE-TECT	E-JECT
DE-POSE	PRO-TECT	RE-JECT
IM-POSE		SUB-JECT(!)
OP-POSE		
PRO-POSE		
RE-POSE		
SUP-POSE		
(PURPOSE!)		

Significantly the word SUB-JECT, like the words PRO-DUCE and PRO-GRESS, can be both a verb and a noun, and when it is a noun the stress will be on the first syllable. The placement of the stress on the root is obviously not a general rule. Seemingly it depends on other factors still to be analyzed into a rule or rules. A good example is the familiar AD-MIRE, an assimilated word from which the longer words

AD-MIR-ABLE AD-MIR-ATION

are derived, the first being an adjective and the second a noun. In neither of these words will the accent fall on the root syllable. But even in these examples, shortness or length of the root word's vowel sound is directly related to the syllable's accented or nonaccented character. In AD-MIRE the I sounds /ī/ and the root syllable carries the accent (the silent E is simply added to indicate the length of the vowel in the root word -MIR-); in the two other words, -MIR- is pronounced with a short /i/ because the syllable carries no accent.

Whatever the rules of accenting in long superstructure words, chances are that the vowel in the stressed syllable will be pronounced long provided that the order of letters in the syllable makes this possible. In the Latinized Greek word

GYM-*NA*-SI-UM

it is the second syllable that is stressed, as in the original tongue. The syllable is -NA-, an open syllable; the pronunciation is nā, the vowel is long.[11] In another example given earlier and syllabized as

E-STAB-LISH-MENT

the stress is, as we would expect, on the root word

STA-BLE

one of those one-and-half syllable words in which the accent naturally falls upon the full syllable. If the root word stands alone its vowel sound is long; the pronunciation is *stā-bl*. The L does not count as a consonant, and the E is silent. However, in the derived verb

E-STAB-LISH

(correctly, it should be syllabized E-STABL-ISH), prosody will not permit a long vowel; the A is short. Nevertheless, it is the root sylla-ble -STABL- that the stress falls on. There is no haphazardness, no irregularity either in spelling or in stress. A second affix, the suffix

-MENT

does not influence the stress on the root syllable. Not so the suffix

-ATION

added to AD-MIRE to make it AD-MIR-ATION. This suffix tries to take over. We can offer it as an almost general rule that in words ending with

-SION   -TION   -OUS   -CIOUS   -TIOUS

the accent is on the next to the last syllable, whether it is long or short. In

AV-AR-I-CIOUS[12]   AD-VEN-TI-TIOUS
TE-LE-VI-SION   CIR-CUM-CI-SION

this syllable is short. In

AD-VAN-TAGE-OUS

it is long, as the silent E indicates. In the words

AD-VEN-TUR-OUS   TREA-CHER-OUS

(is it the R, by any chance?) the rule does not hold: the accent is not on the next to the last syllable. In the many words which end in TION or A-TION, like

N*A*-TION   CO-RON-*A*-TION
AD-MIR-*A*-TION
CON-FIRM-*A*-TION   DE-CLAR-*A*-TION

the stressed vowel has a long sound.

I think that these last three paradigm words are as plain illustra-

tions of the sense and the logic governing English spelling and pronunciation as anyone could wish. Let us first look at the word

AD-MIR-ATION

It should be clear that it is not haphazard irregularity that makes the
root syllable -MIRE (long and accented and pronounced to rhyme
with FIRE) in the verb AD-MIRE change into a short and unstressed
syllable in AD-MIR-A-TION. The rule that the syllable next to the
suffix -TION must be long and stressed is obviously dominant over
any other rule.

The example CON-FIR-MA-TION corroborates this rule. In the
word

CON-FIRM

the stress is on the root syllable. The word is so thoroughly assimilated into the basic English phonic system that its -IR- component
has even assumed the sound /ûr/. But no sooner does the word become compounded into the noun

CON-FIRM-A-TION

than the root syllable becomes unstressed and unassimilated, re-
trieving, so to speak, its old Latin sound *firm.*

Another, even more remarkable example is offered by the sequence

CLEAR   DE-CLARE   DE-CLAR-ATION

three words in which the vowel of the same root syllable is pronounced in three different ways. The root word CLEAR is thoroughly
assimilated from the Latin-French CLARUS/CLAIR. Spoken English assimilated the word as

kleer

and about this there can be no argument. Significantly, of the two
easy choices of a vowel digraph to indicate the sound /ee/, the codifiers of spelling chose EA, not EE, to preserve the A letter of both the
Latin and the French. It is thus for a good reason that the word is
spelled

CLEAR   not   CLEER[13]

In contradistinction, the Germanic word

free

will be spelled FREE, the simplest possible way, not FREA. True, another Germanic word

flee

(meaning a bug) will be spelled FLEA. But this cannot be helped. The simpler spelling FLEE is already occupied by a homophone.

However, as thoroughly assimilated as the word CLEAR may be, when it comes to longer forms, the spelling reverts to the original Latin. The vowel digraph disappears, and the word becomes

DE-CLARE

The root syllable remains long; the stress remains. But even here pronunciation is guided by the rules of phonics, the rule which makes FARE sound like FAIR (*fär*) and to which there can be no exception. But when we finally come to

DE-CLAR-ATION

then even the pronunciation of the root word returns to the original Latin, and at the same time the stress switches to the A in ATION. There is nothing irregular, nothing haphazard in either the spelling or the pronunciation. It all follows from the layered structure of the English language and the split-personality nature of English spelling. Whether one loves or despises the language for it (the German writer Kurt Tucholsky once called English a "conglomeration of foreign words falsely pronounced") makes no difference.

The teacher should not hesitate to teach children to use a dictionary. (There are some good ones prepared for children.) He should not avoid "long" words. There is nothing simpler than to explain to a child of appropriate intelligence that a great many words starting with PRO- (one of those meaningful meaning modifiers) are borrowed from the Latin or Greek, and that this part of the word conveys the idea of "for" or "before" (words starting with PROT- often being an exception). Thus, everyday words such as PRO-BLEM, PRO-DUCE, PRO-FIT, PRO-GRAM, PRO-GRESS, PRO-TECT,[14] and longer words such as PRO-HIB-IT, PRO-MIN-ENT, PRO-MOT-

ER, PRO-FES-SION-AL, PRO-PAG-AN-DA, PRO-NUN-CI-A-TION, are brought closer to understanding. A similar cluster of important everyday words can be grouped around the meaningful meaning modifier EX-. All these words somehow convey the idea of "out of."

In this connection it is possible to draw the brighter child's attention to the fact that *meaningful meaning modifiers usually attach themselves to "learned" words*, or at least assimilated Latin-French words, to what we later shall learn to call "concept" words. *Only concept words are malleable.* In contradistinction, one cannot generally add to basic words any of those sophisticated, Latin or Greek, meaning-changing prefixes or suffixes. *Basic words will accept only simple affixes* of the -LY type, simple meaning modifiers that increase the applicability of words in sentences without essentially affecting their meaning, simple meaning modifiers that (I will emphasize this again) add nothing to the phonic burden. I encourage parents and teachers to make good use of them, to augment a child's reading and expressive vocabulary by familiarizing him with simple meaning modifiers first.

The simplest kinds of dissyllables formed by this type of meaning modifiers I will describe to a child in the lower grades as -ING words" and "-ED words," avoiding, at first, grammatical terminology. Most children know or can simply be told how these suffixes modify meaning. Even the poor reader will learn to handle these suffixes in one lesson. There are no new spelling rules to be observed. It is always the first half of these words that offers the spelling-pronouncing problem, not the ending. Some examples are

SEE/SEE-ING
HEAR/HEAR-ING
BRING/BRING-ING
FIGHT/FIGHT-ING
MAIL/MAIL-ING
FLOW/FLOW-ING
MATE/MAT-ING ⎫
RIDE/RID-ING ⎪
ABIDE/ABID-ING ⎬ (the modifier gets lost)
MOVE/MOV-ING ⎭

BID/BID-DING ⎱ (the last consonant doubles)
FIT/FIT-TING ⎰

WORK-ED ⎫
PLAY-ED ⎪
BOW-ED ⎬ (note the mostly silent E)
MAIL-ED ⎪
FIR-ED ⎪
TIR-ED ⎭

Then come some "-AR words," "-AL words," more "-LY words":

MOL-AR ⎫
POL-AR ⎬ (note the missing silent E)
BRID-AL ⎪
TID-AL ⎭
FREE-LY
GLAD-LY
MAIN-LY
MAN-LY
SICK-LY
STRICT-LY

and finally the comparative-superlative forms (with children, I use the term "grade" forms) of adjectives:

HARD/HARD-ER/HARD-EST
NICE/NIC-ER/NIC-EST (note the missing silent E)
LOW/LOW-ER/LOW-EST

All these words pose no problem once they have been gone over by the teacher and offered to a student who has done the writing-spelling exercises on monosyllables which I outlined earlier. Of course, not all basic words are monosyllables but longer-than-one-syllable basic words offer no specific reading problems, and in two-syllable basic words it is usually the first syllable that poses the problem and is to be solved by the rules of phonics. A few examples, a cluster of "-ER words," should suffice:

FATHER MOTHER SISTER BROTHER
FLOWER FLOUR(!) POWER SOUR(!) PILLAR(!)
COVER CLEVER FEVER(!) CLOVER

BUTTER   MUTTER
LAYER   PRAYER   FIRE(!)   TIRE(!)
ROPER   WAITER   LAW-YER

As the teacher will note, not all of these words are basic words, though some are. FATHER, MOTHER are, in fact, older than Anglo-Saxon. (It would be worth the teacher's and the student's while to look up the origin of these words in an unabridged dictionary.[15]) Others, like

PRAY-ER   WAIT-ER

are derived words and will need further attention. But as far as reading is concerned (I repeat), there is no added challenge.

A peculiar breed of mostly, but not invariably, basic words consists seemingly of one and a half syllables, with the liquid consonant L acting as a kind of semivowel in an always unstressed second syllable. Some examples are

LIT-TLE   BRIT-TLE   CAT-TLE   MET-TLE   BOT-TLE
SCUT-TLE   TI-TLE   TUR-TLE   BRI-DLE   HUR-DLE
   SHUF-FLE   SCUF-FLE   SCRU-PLE STA-BLE

Some of them will accept a prefix,

BE-LITTLE   EN-TITLE   RE-SHUFFLE

like any ordinary one-syllable word or even bloom into a long compounded word like the already quoted

E-STABL-ISH-MENT

In a related group of Latin-French words, a liquid R rather than L figures as a kind of semivowel. The English spell these words in the French manner:

CENTRE   FIBRE   FILTRE

In American English these words are spelled

CEN-TER   FI-BER   FIL-TER

They have become regular two-syllable assimilated words.

NOTES

[1]In a beautiful and moving description of the Metropolitan Museum's exhibition "Harlem On My Mind," a *New York Times* correspondent, Jervis Anderson (*New York Times*, January 26, 1969), used within the confines of a few sentences the following simple and yet evocative verbs (or, rather, participles):

YEARNING STRUGGLING HOPING SPEAKING LOVING
LAUGHING DANCING SINGING SHARING STRIVING

All of their roots (here with a suffix) are, significantly, monosyllables; almost all are spelling problems. A child could learn a fair percentage of English reading rules by just familiarizing himself with the spelling and pronunciation of these ten verbs. Try it! (The word "struggle" is, of course, not quite monosyllabic; it just behaves like one when in the participial form.)

[2]From what I have just said, the reader will anticipate that all these words (verbs, adjectives, nouns) are of Anglo-Saxon origin and so they are, except for ACT and PAIN. But ACT is not really a word denoting some specific kind of doing. It is a more conceptual and, fittingly, a Latin word. As to the word PAIN, it comes through French, also from the Latin. Strangely, the German word SCHMERZ, which has more or less the same meaning, did not make it in English. Its English cognate is SMART, a word much less significative. The exclamation mark after BITTER should, by the way, signify that there is seldom any linguistic rule without exceptions. BITTER is not a monosyllable, though it is basic and Anglo-Saxon. It should finally be noted that some truly basic words

LOVE   PLAY   FIGHT   CRY   HOLD

(in my haphazard collection) are nouns and verbs at the same time.

[3]There is no reason why a child in elementary school should not learn something about this structured nature of the English language, about its mainly Germanic (and older) ground structure (the monosyllables with the phonics problems), the Normanic-French in-between layer and the Latin-Greek superstructure. An English-speaking child will appreciate his language more if he is shown these layered differences since they are so conspicuous. For example, compare the two rows of words:

OX   CALF   SHEEP   SOW   DEER

BEEF   VEAL   MUTTON   PORK   VENISON

The upper are older and Germanic words: the lower are later and French words. They are related in pairs but still mean different things; Beef is the meat of the ox, veal that of the calf, etc. The French words were obviously used in the kitchen. (For a Marxist historian such a detail could be of some interest. Most likely cowherds, shepherds, and servants were Anglo-Saxon while the royal household was run by their Norman-French conquerors.) Why not tell such things to students while they learn their phonics on SHEEP, BEEF, VEAL, etc.?

[4]AB, for example, signifies "away."

[5]Earlier, I referred to this part as the "meaning-giving" syllable, and to the prefix as a "meaning modifier." I also discussed some of the problems of stress or accent which the teacher might find worth repeating.

[6]This happens to be an original Latin word, now fully assimilated into the English spelling system.

[7]Today the vocabulary of even the semiliterate is replete with concept words (about which see the next chapter). Which words belong to "basic" English depends mainly on the viewpoint of the compiler. One justifiable viewpoint would be that only words of Anglo-Saxon origin are "basic" words (OX, yes; BEEF, no). If "basic" means the vocabulary in everyday use among average people, then our English is, indeed, highly conceptualized, and only partially Anglo-Saxon.

[8]Only "almost." Some of the rules of retroactive modification have spilled over into their domain. Also accent sometimes modifies the sound value of a vowel (for examples, see p. 94).

[9]A great many so-called irregularities of English spelling, accenting, and pronunciation would be found to follow a logical course if this circumstance were paid due attention. Words like POLICE, DEMISE, or GARAGE are, as I have pointed out, not "irregularly" accented or pronounced. They are French words, with the vowels pronounced in the French manner and the accent on the last syllable. They are unassimilated, unincorporated, relatively new, still essentially foreign words. (Those who call the POLICE *polīs* on account of some spelling analogy to the Germanic word LOUSE/ LICE reveal their ignorance when they make this "joke.") As I stressed in the earlier part of this essay, the French silent E retroacts upon the immediately preceding consonant and *not*, like its English counterpart, upon the preceding vowel. It is not exceptional, not an irregularity, that POLICE is pronounced *polees* instead of *polīs*.

[10]I realize that spellings could be CATA-LOGUE, PRO-GRAMME, etc. With the young American student in mind, I rather choose the simpler version.

[11]This will be a good occasion for the student to learn a new phonics rule, one of the rules of prosody, using the word GYMNASIUM as paradigm:

1. *A vowel followed by two consonants* (for example, GYMN-) *tends to be short.*

2. *A vowel followed by one consonant* (for example, NAS-) *or no consonant* (example, -SI-) *can be long or short* as the case may be (often depending on where the accent falls).

[12]We will again try to find some sense, some accordance with rules. AVARI-CIOUS comes from the unassimilated French AVARICE, in which (as in POLICE) the silent E merely serves as a modifier of the C, in the French manner. Hence, the correct pronunciation is

avaris

not

avaris

(with the accent on the last syllable) and the derived adjective sounds

avarishuz

with the accent on the next to the last syllable, as the rule requires.

[13]Except in CHANTICLEER or CHAUNTECLEER. But this has its own literary-historical reasons.

[14]The placement of the accent in this particular cluster of words once more indicates that the question is in need of much more refined analysis: PRO-BLEM and PRO-GRAM are stressed on the first syllable and are nouns, PRO-TECT is stressed on the second syllable and is a verb, PRO-DUCE and PRO-GRESS can be stressed on either syllable and are nouns in one case and verbs in the other, but PRO-FIT is always stressed on the first syllable whether noun or verb.

[15]As an item of interest I should mention, since Webster's *Third New International Dictionary*, Unabridged, has missed it, that in Hebrew

$$\bar{a}hv \text{ is FATHER}$$
$$\bar{a}m \text{ is MOTHER}$$

while in Hungarian the words are spelled APA and ANYA. Thus, the "deciding consonants" *P-F-V* and *M-N* are the same or similar in languages as different as Greek, English, Hebrew, and Hungarian.

CHAPTER SIX

The Birth of Concepts and the Metamorphosis of Concepts — The Triplet PEACE/AP-PEASE/AP-PEASE-MENT — "And the RAIN IT RAINETH" (Shakespeare) — Examples of Concepts Built on Concepts: The Quadruplet RE-FRIGER-AT(E)-OR — The Difference Between AN-NOUNCE-MENT and AN-NUNCI-AT(E)-ION

I broke off my first rather cursory discussion of compounded words (words amplified by a prefix or suffix or both) after presenting one of my favorite examples, the word

BE-NIGHT-ED

I did not at that time enter into any kind of analysis of what the prefix or suffix does to the word, though for the enrichment of both the understood and spelled vocabulary it is essential to explain to the student what these added syllables actually are for. All I said at that time was that, to a student familiar with the phonics of the root word -NIGHT-, this "long" word offers no new reading (sound solving) challenge.

Some pages later I added that actually the longer a compounded word, the easier the job, chances are, in reading it. Compounded words like

BE-LOV(E)-ED   RE-CEIV-ER

PRO-CEED-INGS   DIS-HEART-ENING

(the first and the last have Anglo-Saxon "basic" roots, the two others are built around "assimilated" Latin-French roots) continue to carry their problem load of phonics in their respective root words. In rather sharp contrast superstructure words like

OVER-POPUL-ATION   IN-CINER-ATOR
TRANS-CEND-ENT-AL-ISM   AMPHI-THE-A-TER
HELIC-O-PTER[1]

offer no problem features. *There are no retroactive modifiers, no silent letters, no capricious digraphs in long Latin (or Greek) words!* They can be read (phonetically, as I said) as soon as some very easy general rules or peculiarities of pronunciation have been learned or memorized. (Some of these have already been mentioned, e.g., the peculiar sound equivalents of the suffixes

-SION   -TION   -IOUS   -TIOUS

and the placement of the stress on the preceding syllable. Another such rule is that PH sounds like /f/ in "learned" words.)

In fact, as I showed in the previous chapter by several rather attractive examples (I used the words FIRM and CLEAR as paradigms), a root word might well be weighted down with phonic problems as long as it is part of a half-long word but will revert to the less complicated Latin spelling and pronunciation as it gets to be part of a longer superstructure word.

Another good example is a word like

LABOR

a Latin word with the stress on the first syllable. As we might expect, the sound of this syllable has become a long /ā/ in English, and a prefix or suffix will not change this as long as the stress remains on the same syllable, as, e.g., in

BE-LABOR   LABOR-ITE   LABOR-ER

But take the somewhat longer

LABOR-IOUS

an adjective derived by adding the suffix -IOUS. According to the rule given earlier, this suffix is wont to pull the accent over to the preceding syllable. Thus, in LABORI-OUS the stress is not on the first syllable LA- any longer. It has shifted to the second syllable and the A becomes a short vowel, something like /a/ in WOMAN. The same will also hold for the word

LABOR-ATORY

pronounced in England with the stress on the second syllable.

But this is not the whole story. In the words

E-LABOR-ATE (adjective)

and

E-LABOR-ATE (verb)

the accent falls on the first syllable of the root. In spite of this, the vowel reverts to its original Latin sound. In

E-LABOR-ATION[2]

the accent, according to rule, falls on the A of the suffix. But the root word again retains the sound of the original Latin. Obviously these have become superstructure words, and superstructure words tend to retain their original Latin sound character.

All this follows strict rules. They just have to be found and taught. Nothing is haphazard.

I shall continue with a somewhat more complex word, also one of my favorite teaching examples.[3] The word is

AP-PEASE-MENT

another of these easy long words with one "meaning-giving," stressed, and (more often than not) long-voweled syllable, plus two short-voweled, unstressed "meaning-adjusting" syllables, a prefix and a suffix. Lacking a better term, I shall refer to compound words structured in this manner as "triplet" verbs, nouns, etc. I might just as well use this word to demonstrate the way I make my student-patients approach this type of compounded word.

It would never occur to anyone to present a word like

AP-PEASE-MENT

as a "package," as a word to be memorized visually as the symbol of a concept, the way adherents of the "meaning" technique would necessarily have to handle it, if words of such length and structure were included in their "planned" vocabulary. The word is too difficult. The look-and-say approach breaks down in the face of words of this complexity, not to mention still longer, still more complex, truly superstructure words. Obviously, poor readers, poorly taught poor readers, poor readers taught by the look-and-say method, must feel almost bewildered by such "long" words. "I have not yet had that word" or "I have never seen that word" is much too often heard as a conditioned response even to much shorter words. How can they ever be expected to memorize such a complex word? When I use the adjective "easy" in connection with "long" (or "longer") words, I mean that the embellishments, the prefixes and suffixes which make the words long, don't really add to the difficulty of "sounding" them if (and only if) the child has been brought up on the "code" (or "de-coding") approach.

It must be hard enough for a child to commit to memory a nonfamily "concept" word like PEACE ("Why not PEES?" asked one of my young patients); it must be utterly impossible to commit a word like APPEASEMENT to memory, whatever the number of repetitions.

In my session with a student-patient I first ascertain whether the *spelled word*

PEACE

is one familiar to him. (I hope that at least the "concept" is! It should be among the two to four thousand words a first-grader is supposed to know when he hears them!) If it is not (i.e., if he cannot read the word), then I try to approach it along some of the phonics routes presented earlier. By one or another of them even the poorest reader will finally be brought to recognize that the spelled word PEACE represents the sound word

pees

and if the "concepts" *pees* (of luggage) and *pees* (on earth) are both[4] known to him, he can finally be brought to attach the proper concept to the proper pattern.

I will then ascertain whether my young patient is able to attack the spelled word,

AP-PEASE

(Again the "concept" should be familiar to a boy nine or ten years old who comes from a middle-class family even if the printed word is one he has "not yet learned.") I used the word to show that English spelling does its best to indicate pronunciation whenever possible, in spite of all the traditionalism that so often burdens it. The word

AP-PEASE (pronounced *ap-peez*)

is obviously related to the root word

PEACE (pronounced *pees*)

but the spoken word AP-PEASE contains a /z/ sound which cannot be represented in English spelling by the letter C. Hence the spelling has necessarily changed: an S replaces the root word's C.[5]

However, all these details are merely minor items in phonics, warmed over, and not the reason why I think it worthwhile to tarry with the word AP-PEASE. It is my feeling that with a paradigm of this type a student can take an important step toward the enrichment of his conceptual vocabulary. More specifically, a word like AP-PEASE can make him understand the significance of a prefix, a "meaning-modifier" syllable, attached to the front of a root word for the purpose of constructing a related but still new concept. The job of prefixes (also, of course, of suffixes) is to help in the creation of related but still new and more complex concepts. While the word PEACE can and must be attacked by phonics (it is an "incorporated" Latin-French word), reading a word like AP-PEASE involves more than phonics. It involves an analytical process, a taking apart, the process of finding in a word a part to which the laws of phonic attack apply (the root word) and some other part or parts where such an attack is unnecessary. The word AP-PEASE contains an obvious root word and a syllable attached to its front end (a prefix), a syllable which modulates both the meaning and (this is an important item previously mentioned cursorily) the grammatical standing of the original root word without, in essence, changing the meaning. When we say AP-PEASE, we are talking about something related to PEACE.

But what does the expression "grammatical standing" mean? The concept needs some careful analysis.

PEACE is a noun, the name of a concept: AP-PEASE is a verb, the name of an action, of an action related to the concept symbolized by the noun. PEACE is a *noun concept* and the job of this particular prefix AD- (AP- is merely a euphonistic modification of the prefix AD-) is to change it into an *action concept*, a *verb concept*, specifically, a "direction-expressing" verb. (AD in Latin is both a preposition and a prefix. Either way it denotes direction. AD ASTRA means "Toward the stars.")

Attaching another syllable, the suffix -MENT, to the other end of this newly created word reverts the verb concept into a *noun concept*. This new word still relates to the concept PEACE and still refers to the directed action AP-PEASE, but its grammatical standing is once again that of a noun concept. It is this change, the change of the word from verb to noun that permits us to make further statements about the action in a grammatically correct fashion, statements which might otherwise be linguistically impossible. We can say about PEACE that IT is "good," "eternal," "unobtainable," etc., because, according to the rules of grammar, it is a noun. We can say about AP-PEASE-MENT that IT is "bad," "necessary," "unavoidable," or that IT won't work, all because it is a noun. We can, in other words, use pronouns *for* it and predicates *with* it, but, to repeat, we can do this only because, with the suffix -MENT, we turned our action concept back into a concept noun. The job of the suffix -MENT is to change concept verbs into concepts nouns without change of meaning.

I have just used the phrases "in a grammatically correct fashion" and "which would otherwise be linguistically impossible." The latter is, in fact, somewhat too sweeping a statement. A short digression from our actual topic will be necessary to qualify it.

As far as I can tell, all Western and Oriental linguistic civilizations require that a concept be given grammatical noun form, the grammatical form of a "thing," before any statement can be made about it. But as the great American linguist Benjamin Whorf discovered, this is not an a priori necessity, not the only possible way of communication. *We* say THE RAIN FALLS or, referring to RAIN, that IT FALLS: we can also say that "IT" RAINS, meaning THE RAIN RAINS: we can even say with Shakespeare *(Twelfth Night)* that THE RAIN IT RAINETH. We can do all this because we have made RAIN a "thing." We can make a statement about it (use it as the subject of a predicate verb), and we can use a pronoun for it. But this is not true, for instance, of the Hopi language which Whorf studied. The Hopi have no noun for the concept RAIN. To their way of thinking RAIN is not a thing but a happening. You cannot, in their language, say about RAIN that it does NOT FALL or that IT STOPPED. RAIN "is" not, that is, it does not exist, when it does not FALL.

Bolinger (1968) uses the example

(the) WIND BLOWS

to illustrate Whorf's concepts. One must assume that the Hopi have no noun for WIND either and a child's question would be justified: "What does the WIND do when it does not BLOW?"

Volume III (1968) of the *Perspectives* published by *Encyclopaedia Brittanica*, contains an excellent two-page summary on Whorf's ideas. (I recommend reading it.) I must quote one sentence:

"The Hopi think of reality mainly in terms of *events*, eschewing the emphasis upon subject and predicate built into Indo-European language and thought."

It should be worthwhile pointing out, in this connection, to both the teacher and the student of the English language that, in English, RAIN (like LOVE) is both a noun and a verb. One does not even need a prefix, as in PEACE, or a change of letter, as in ADVICE, to transform one into the other. This, to my mind, indicates that, even if only in some not fully conscious manner, the English language also suggests that RAINING (like LOVING) is less a thing than it is a happening. This gives us two degrees of freedom: we can make statements about a "subject" RAIN (it can be "welcome," "too little," "torrential"); we can also modulate a "verb" RAIN (it RAINED, it will RAIN, etc.).

By the way, the French and the Germans also use IT (a neuter pronoun) as subject, with RAINS as the predicate, to describe the happening IT RAINS = IL PLEUT = ES REGNET. They, too, just cannot bear a predicate without a grammatical subject.

While this, admittedly, is an abstruse subject, I feel that I am not unjustified in mentioning it in this chapter. We shall all better understand our Indo-European mode of thinking, concept forming, and communication if we realize that (like our calendar and our algorithm) it too has its "history," that it is in the final analysis also based on "consensus," and that other modes of thinking and communicating, quite different from ours, are not only possible but have in fact developed and come to fruition. Not that there is anything wrong with our Indo-European way of thinking. Our technique of *nominalizing actions*, our being able to turn AP-PEASE, an act, into AP-PEASE-MENT, a grammatical noun, about which more general statements can be made, is in my view, one of the sublime achievements of our concept-based civilization and, ultimately, and with due credit to the French, one of the glories of the English language. I guess the Hopi are, in a way, worse off by not being able to nominalize RAIN and WIND.

The suffix -MENT is, of course, not the only one that will turn a verb concept into a noun concept. One can add, for example, the suffix -ER instead of -MENT to AP-PEASE, when one is again presented with a noun, a different kind of derived concept noun. The word

$$\text{AP-PEAS(E)-ER}$$

signifies a person who is identified by what he does: *he* AP-PEASES.

In the example

$$\text{AD-VICE } \textit{(advis)} \qquad \text{AD-VISE } \textit{(adviz)}$$

(they are both derived words having been formed with the prefix AD-) one of the changes in grammatical standing is achieved simply by a change of sound: AD-VICE is a noun concept, AD-VISE (to give AD-VICE) is a verb concept. The verb is pronounced with a /z/ at the end, and this must be indicated.[6] Again, we can add the suffix -MENT and have the new noun concept

AD-VISE-MENT

or we can add the suffix -ER and have the noun concept

AD-VIS(E)-ER[7]

denoting a person who AD-VISES, who gives AD-VICE.

In the example

BELIEF   BELIEVE[8]

it is again the shift of a final consonant sound (in this instance from /f/ to /v/) which indicates the change in grammatical standing, and only the suffix -ER seems to be fitting.[9] Again the suffix is added to the verb, not to the noun, to form the derived concept noun,

BELIEV(E)-ER

A word like

BELIEF-ER

would make no sense. The term BELIEV(E)-ER describes one who BELIEVES, not his BELIEF, just as the term AD-VISER denotes the person who ADVISES, not his ADVICE. Words like

ADVIC(E)-ER   ADVICE-MENT

would make no sense. The ending -ER, like the ending -MENT, always attaches itself to an action word, a verb concept; it signifies a person, or a DEVICE (not a DEVISE) that carries out an action.

VOT(E)-ER   COM-PUT(E)-ER

are added examples for the two alternatives. Both are action-derived nouns or, even more specifically, nouns that *name a person or a thing* (e.g., a machine) *in terms of what he, or it, does.* VOT(E)-ER is a person who votes (will vote, can vote, has voted, etc.) COM-PUT(E)-ER is a machine that computes.

But let me return to my earlier example,

PEACE/APPEASE/AP-PEASE-MENT

a triplet of related meanings arrived at by way of first modulating a noun into a verb and then this derived verb into a noun again, into what I call a triplet noun.

An important restriction should be established before we encourage a student to build word triplets as if they were playing a game of scrabble. The student must come to realize that it is only with words like PEACE, ADVICE, BELIEF that meaning can be modulated. He must come to realize that no such games can be played with, say, the word

AP-PLE

because this word is a sound symbol for (the name of) a *thing*.[10] It does not stand for a *concept* and AP- is not a prefix. *Names of things cannot be modulated, only names of concepts.*

Once the student has understood the structural problems in new concept formation, hundreds of new words are open to him without his ever bothering with memorizing. A scrabble game with, say, variable prefix and unchanging suffix can give such triplets as

SIGN	AS-SIGN	AS-SIGN-MENT
RANGE	AR-RANGE	AR-RANGE-MENT
RANGE	DE-RANGE	DE-RANGE-MENT
CITE	EX-CITE	EX-CITE-MENT
COURAGE	EN-COURAGE	EN-COURAGE-MENT
RICH	EN-RICH	EN-RICH-MENT
FRESH	RE-FRESH	RE-FRESH-MENT

all of them words which it is almost impossible to memorize by any look-and-say technique but which are easily "solved" and understood when built up or analyzed by the modified phonics method I encourage. Whether the student knows these words or these concepts does not matter at the moment. Most students will be familiar with most of them.

The ubiquitousness of compounded verb concepts and noun concepts in our language is almost unbelievable. There cannot be a boy who is eight or nine years old, in a middle-class American family, who has not come across any number of situations involving them. For example, his parents may leave for his older brother or sister's

COM-MENCE-MENT

They are happy because his marks show

IM-PROVE-MENT

They send out

AN-NOUNCE-MENTS

to let friends know about his older sister's

EN-GAGE-MENT[11]

There cannot be a boy, even in a family with restricted vocabulary, who will not have heard in Sunday School about the Ten

COM-MAND-MENTS

or in class about the

DE-CLAR-ATION (of) IN-DE-PEND-ENCE

two noun concepts ending in other kinds of suffixes. The last of them is a "quadruplet" noun, formed from a triplet noun,

DE-PEND-ENCE

by a pre-prefix IN- which negates the meaning of the triplet concept noun.
It is just as unlikely that our boy will never have heard the teacher talk about the

(American) CON-STITU-TION

or the

(Federal) GOVERN-MENT

the latter a "doublet" noun, if I may so call it, formed from an anglicized Latin verb concept, GOVERN, which is not a derived word itself.

The chances are that even the poorest reader will know a great number of concept words when he hears them. I am quite sure that, of the two thousand or four thousand heard words, spoken words, an average American child is expected to know in the first grade, a fair percentage are concept words. By the time the child is in the second or third grade, he must have added hundreds of other concept words. He must know what

PRE-SENT	AB-SENT
AD-DI-TION	SUB-TRAC-TION,
VAC-ATION	RE-GIST(E)R-ATION,
RE-LIGION	PRAY-ER
TEACH-ER	PRINCIP-AL,

PUBLIC   PAROCH-IAL
CLASS-ROOM   PLAY-GROUND[12]

mean, and if he does not, chances are that he is culturally and socially deprived, and not dyslexic.

The tragedy is that a child, if he is a retarded reader, never has a chance even to see these words which he "must not be exposed to" (though they are most likely familiar to him), and which are much easier to handle than most of the words in the stories with scientifically restricted vocabulary to which he is constantly exposed. Let me once more jot down some of the words I have just listed in a haphazard manner. I shall capitalize the root words, those parts of the compounded concept nouns that carry both the meaning and the "phonic burden":

com-MENCE-ment
im-PROVE-ment
an-NOUNCE-ment
en-GAGE-ment
a-PART-ment
a-MUSE-ment
com-MAND-ment
de-CLAR-ation
in-de-PEND-ence
con-STITU-tion
GOVERN-ment

To a child who has learned the simple phonic rules about the silent E and the E as modifier of C and G, who has learned to guess the sound value of an occasional digraph (there are practically no digraphs in long concept words!), and who has even a vague idea about how the letter R plays tricks with preceding vowels, none of these root words will offer any difficulty. It is so much harder to read "family" words like

HAIR   HEART   HEAR   HEAD   HARE
HARD   FACE   FAKE   GIRL   FIRM

Let us once more look at the word

IN-DE-PEND-ENCE

It reveals, in such an elegant manner, the devious ways of concepts. The root word is the Latin (French)

PEND(ere) = to hang

a verb from which comes another verb,

DE-PEND

a concept word in verb form denoting the fact that something (or somebody) is conditioned by (originally "hanging from") something (or somebody). This verb concept can be transformed into a noun concept

DE-PEND-ENCE

by adding the Latin (French) suffix -ENCE. And this brings us back to

IN-DE-PEND-ENCE

the negation of DE-PEND-ENCE. What a beautiful way to express a thought!

This suffix -ENCE or -ENCY can be added to a large class of concept verbs to make concept nouns. The same verbs can also be given the status of adjectives, or of nouns with a different meaning, a modified meaning, by adding the suffix -ENT.

This makes it possible to state that someone is

DE-PEND-ENT (on)
IN-DE-PEND-ENT (of)
(a) DE-PEND-ENT (of)

somebody (something) else. This kind of analysis will again add scores of words, concept words, previously avoided words, to a reader's vocabulary, words that pose no spelling problems whatever. The following examples will suffice:

PRES-ENT/PRES-ENCE
PRE-SID-ENT/PRE-SID-ENCY
COR-RE-SPOND-ENT/COR-RE-SPOND-ENCE
EF-FICI-ENT/EF-FICI-ENCY

The related suffixes

-ANT   -ANCE   -ANCY

which also came to us through the French, give us more, easily read, easily spelled pairs of words, such as

AS-SIST-ANT/AS-SIST-ANCE
DOMIN-ANT/DOMIN-ANCE
VAC-ANT/VAC-ANCY

As we see in some of the last examples, the ending of the compounded nouns can be one of several suffixes, the root word need not be a noun, the triplet need not be a noun, and the triplet form is not a *sine-qua-non*. Flexibility and variability add greatly to the enrichment of our conceptual vocabulary.

We have just had the word DE-PEND-ENT, a compounded triplet word, with the grammatical standing of an adjective or noun. Another compounded word from the same root is

DE-PEND-ABLE

a triplet adjective with a different suffix. Rather than adding random examples ending in the same suffix, I want to make just one point: In the compounded adjectives

TRACE-ABLE   PEACE-ABLE

we find our familiar silent E filling some of its regular jobs. They are added examples to show how circumspect English spelling can be in indicating pronunciation as accurately as feasible. Silent E's are not usually retained in the middle of words. Here we have some exceptions, exceptions serving a good purpose.

We have already met another kind of concept adjective,

LABOR-IOUS

formed by the suffix

-IOUS

We can add

IL-LUST(E)R-IOUS   INDU-STR(U)-IOUS

as examples of compounded adjectives formed by the same suffix. Other examples of compounded adjectives with different suffixes are

VOCA-TION-AL
INDU-STR(U)-IAL
CON-STRUCT-IVE
AD-HES-IVE

The adjective concept

AC-CID-ENT-AL[13]

is structurally a quadruplet adjective concept formed with the -AL suffix from the triplet noun concept

AC-CID-ENT

The adjective concept

NAT-ION-AL[14]

is one certainly familiar to youngsters of any background and so, probably, is the adjective

INTER-NAT-ION-AL

I don't have sufficient experience to tell how soon this type of word can be introduced into the reading vocabulary of a child. There is obviously no point trying to force the readings of words that have no place yet in the child's spoken concept vocabulary. There must be tremendous differences due to different backgrounds. I had a pastor's son as a patient who, in spite of being a poor reader, was familiar with the adjective concept

INTER-DE-NOMIN-ATION-AL

which he could explain to me intelligently. Long as this word is, the written word offers no reading problem as soon as it is sounded according to my phonic and analytic technique. I must, of course, stress again that I don't for a moment suggest the analysis of such a long and complex word as a paradigm. Still, in this case I used this rather involved word as an example to show how complex English words are actually structured. I built a kind of "Christmas tree" of words, starting at the top, with the meaning-giving part as the (capitalized) trunk and the meaning-modifying prefixes and suffixes as siding branches:

NOMEN	root noun (Latin)
NOMIN-are	root verb (Latin)
NOMIN-ate	derived verb
NOMIN-ation	noun from verb
de-NOMIN-ation	noun from noun
de-NOMIN-ation-al	adjective from noun
inter-de-NOMIN-ation-al[15]	adjective from adjective

This was a great success. From then on, the boy was no longer afraid of those "impossible" long words.

In contradistinction to such long words,

MOVE	MENT
GOVERN	MENT
CIT(E)	ATION
TU	TOR
TUI	TION
TESTA	MENT

are examples of short noun concepts formed in a single step from the respective root verbs MOVE, GOVERN, and CITE and the Latin roots for GUARD (or TEACH) and for BEING WITNESS.

The doublet earlier given

LABOR/BE-LABOR

is an example of a root word and the prefix BE- forming a concept verb. There is no further step. It should be noted that LABOR, which can be both a noun and a verb, is a verb in this instance. Only verbs can accept the prefix BE- to add momentum to the root verb. All the words we have used in an earlier cluster of examples

BE-COME   BE-GET   etc.

are verbs. (Even HEAD in BE-HEAD is!)

Any adjective can be transformed into a concept noun by the suffix -NESS, e.g.,

KIND/KINDNESS

into a noun about which statements can be made as if the quality were a thing. Another example of such a derived noun is

GRACIOUS-NESS

What at first glance appears to be a root adjective is, of course, itself already a derived word.

CHILD-HOOD

is a strange concept word, a noun formed from a noun. It turns a concrete term into an abstract one.

The two short noun concepts

JUDGE-MENT   JUDGE-SHIP

offer further insight into the ways concepts are formed. The root word JUDGE, like the word LABOR, happens to be both a verb and noun. In the combination

JUDGE-MENT

(also, and for no good reason, spelled JUDG-MENT) the root word must obviously be considered a verb. As I have emphasized repeatedly, it is *verbs* which, through the addition of the meaning-modifying suffix -MENT, change their grammatical standing to nouns. Whether we say of the JUDGE-MENT of Paris that it was fateful or foolish, we still talk about an act, about the JUDG(E)-ING. In contradistinction when we deal with the word

JUDGE-SHIP

we are not dealing with any act of JUDGE-MENT. We are actually forming a noun concept from another noun concept, from the noun

JUDGE, a noun that refers to a person whom we find properly identi-fied ("named") by what he does. What the compounded noun con-cept JUDGE-SHIP aims at is abstracting the office, the dignity, the occupation of such an individual from his person. The suffix -SHIP enables us to make a statement about the office, the dignity, the occu-pation itself, independent of the person holding it. Other similar words, quite well understood even by the unsophisticated, are

AP-PRENTICE-SHIP
PENMAN-SHIP

The first noun is compounded from a triplet noun, AP-PRENT-ICE (with the French-inspired ending -ICE, pronounced *is*); the second comes from PENMAN, a simple compound noun. Both words identify a person in terms of what he does.

Some paragraphs earlier I gave a few examples of nouns ending in -ER and nam-ing a person or a device in terms of what he or it does. Another group of everyday words of similar structure and with similar connotations should also be mentioned. They are formed with the suffix -OR (originally Latin). The example TUT-OR (TU-TOR) has already been cited; the word

RE-FRIGER-AT(E)-OR

will now be analyzed as a paradigm. It is actually a quadruplet word. It is formed from the Latin root for "freezing." The prefix RE- (something being done regularly, repeat-edly) merely serves as a reinforcement; the suffix -ATE produces a verb concept which offers two possible ways to form a complex noun concept with a subsuffix

-ION   or   -OR

In the first case, we again have a nominalized action word,

RE-FRIGER-AT(E)-ION

In the second case we have the noun

RE-FRIGER-AT(E)-OR

which denotes a device that does just that: it

RE-FRIGER-ATEs[16]

Our conceptualized language is replete with these types of verb concepts and action-derived noun concepts. They are usually new words relating to our technical civilization. They do not come through French but have a direct Latin root and are so common that the language has produced special phonic rules for their pronunciation.

in the case of the action-expressing noun RE-FRIGER-AT(E)-ION, the suffix -ATE and the subsuffix -ION coalesce into one syllable, which is always stressed and sounds *āshn*. In the case of the device-denoting word RE-FRIGER-AT(E)-OR, the suffix and subsuffix are pronounced as two syllables and the accent is usually on the root word. An average American child knows scores of such words. Other examples are the quadruplets

AN-NUNCI-AT(E)-ION   PRO-NUNCI-AT(E)-ION

They show that the alternate noun formations need not always be realized. I have never seen the theoretically correct word forms

AN-NUNCI-ATOR[17]   PRO-NUNCI-ATOR

used.

    There are instances where the root word has been lost from actual English parlance (one has to recover it from the dictionary), though the essential triplet or sometimes quadruplet structure is retained. Examples are

A-GREE	A-GREE-MENT
AD-VERTISE	AD-VERTISE-MENT
AN-NOUNCE	AN-NOUNCE-MENT, AN-NUNCI-ATION
PRO-NOUNCE	PRO-NOUNCE-MENT, PRO-NUNCI-ATION
COM-MAND	COM-MAND-MENT
IN-STINCT	IN-STINCT-IVE
CON-STRUCT	CON-STRUCT-IVE
IN-STRUCT	IN-STRUCT-OR, IN-STRUC(T)-TION
IN-STITUTE	IN-STITU-TION

    A word like

IN-STRU-MENT

is by now almost a concrete noun, the name of a thing. One can "play" it. (It would, I guess, almost qualify for the look-and-say vocabulary.) Both of the first steps in the formation of what actually is a triplet are practically lost.

    The same holds for the word

AC-CID-ENT

mentioned earlier. It is a true triplet but by now so strongly welded that both the root word (Latin, CADere) and the first derivative word (Latin, AC-CIDere) have disappeared from usage. None of the triplet character has gotten lost in the compounded word that inevitably comes to mind:

IN-SUR(E)-ANCE

The teacher should miss no occasion to show how English spelling tries its best to be a reliable aid of pronunciation. In the spoken verbs

AN-NOUNCE   PRO-NOUNCE

as well as in the spoken nouns

AN-NOUNCE-MENT   PRO-NOUNCE-MENT
AN-NOUNC(E)-ER

we encounter a diphthong in the root word. By its very nature, a diphthong has a "long vowel" value. In the spelled words we find a vowel digraph, accordingly. And, of course, -NOUNCE, the root word, carries the stress. In

AN-NUNCI-ATION   PRO-NUNCI-ATION

the very structure of the words places the stress on the A of -ATION. This is a "rule," not an irregularity. Thus, the root word becomes unstressed and, as is properly indicated by the spelling, its vowel becomes short.

Here the teacher could also refer to the example

CLEAR/DE-CLAR-ATION

in the previous chapter. (It is essential that, by repetition, by cross-referencing, the student be constantly made aware of the prevalence of rules, of the reassuring reign of logic in English spelling.) The parallels are obvious: -NOUNCE-, like CLEAR, is an assimilated word whose spelling is governed by the phonic rules of basic English.[18] In contrast, AN-NUNCI-ATION, like DE-CLAR-ATION, reverts to the exact spelling of the Latin. Both are superstructure words.

In this particular example there is another, hidden significance: We see that in the two word pairs, AN-NOUNCE-MENT, AN-NUNCI-ATION vs. PRO-NOUNCE-MENT, PRO-NUNCI-ATION, only one member of each pair retains the root in its -NOUNCE- form. As I previously pointed out, the suffix -MENT does nothing but change a verb concept into a grammatical noun form to permit handling of it. It is therefore to be expected that it is the noun forms ending in -MENT which retain the more purely verbal nature of the concepts. What a fine and beautiful distinction! We can describe the biblical *event* or the innumerable paintings of which it is the subject, as

AN-NUNCI-ATION

and may say that the Angel Gabriel made an

AN-NOUNCE-MENT

thus referring to the very *act* of AN-NOUNC(E)-ING. But we cannot use the words the other way around. We cannot call the event an AN-NOUNCE-MENT, and we cannot say that the Angel made an AN-NUNCI-ATION. The two words are not interchangeable synonyms. The latter describes an "event," a "situation," and the former an "act." Nothing, as one can see, is haphazard in these spellings, nothing irregular. It is all so rich, so meaningful, so exquisitely planned. One must love the English language for it!

NOTES

[1] I must repeat that I do not expect eight- or nine-year-old boys to understand these words (except possibly the last or the second). But if they have been taught well, they should be able to phoneticize the words without much difficulty. Also it must be repeated that I do not follow any phonetic system in syllabication. I try, for didactic purposes, to keep prefixes and suffixes visually separated from the root (or should it be called the "body"?) of compounded words (IN-CINER-ATOR or IN-CINER-AT(E)-OR). I also try to indicate the components of compound words (HELIC-O-PTER or HELICO-PTER, not HELI-COPTER).

[2] Words ending in -ATION actually carry a suffix, -ATE, and a subsuffix, -ION, fused into one. Both are direct takeovers from Latin without apparent Norman-French intercessors.

[3] There is some repetition in this discussion. It was as a result of a lesson given to a bright poor reader that the idea of this whole exposition was born, and I record here part of that lesson almost verbatim. During that session the role of prefixes and suffixes became clear to me. To me this was rewarding insight; to the patient-student it was a revelation; to a linguist it must all be old stuff.

[4] There actually exists a third homophone, *pees* = PEAS, the plural of PEA.

[5] A similar explanation will get a child over the hurdle of the common spelling confusion between

ADVICE   ADVISE
DEVICE   DEVISE

both derived words from the Latin root for VISION.

[6] A teacher with love and respect for the English language (and a sensitive ear!) will here, however timidly, again point out some possible "rule." Here is the word pair

CHOOSE and CHOICE, of French origin and assimilated. Isn't it interesting (she might interject) that again the verb is spelled with an "S," here pronounced as /z/, and the noun with C, which cannot be pronounced as a /z/? Here is another example (she might add) of the fact, that, whenever possible, English spelling does choose the spelling alternative that better indicates pronunciation.

[7]Here again, the teacher can point out how careful, wise, and circumspect English spelling actually is. In the word ADVISE, the silent word-concluding E indicates pronunciation accurately. The addition of the suffix -MENT pushes the syllable -VISE into the center of the word, but the pronunciation indicator is retained. When the suffix itself happens to begin with an E, there is no need to retain the silent E and the correct spelling is ADVISER.

[8]Note also the words

GRIEF   GRIEVE

SHELF   SHELVE

to see that we are dealing with trends, not haphazard unplanned arrangements. By the way, why

BELIEVE   GRIEVE   SHELVE

are spelled with a silent E when their noun partners are not, I don't know. But it is a "rule."

[9]The word BELIEVE-MENT does not exist. It would add nothing to what BELIEF already says. English is beautifully flexible in this respect. A word that is not needed is never born. There are many words in the English dictionary, but not too many.

[10]I assume that for APPLE even the Hopi will have a noun.

[11]I hardly dare to mention such words as

A-PART-MENT   A-MUSE-MENT

What child will not know them? (It is in the area of familiar "long" words that cultural and language deprivation so sorely manifest themselves in our urban slums.)

[12]The last two are actually compound and not compounded or derived words.

[13]The ending -AL in

AC-CID-ENT-AL

could properly be called a sub-suffix. The prefix IN- in

IN-DE-PEND-ENCE

is a pre-prefix.

[14]The word

NAT-ION-AL

is, of course, not a triplet adjective in the sense in which I have, for our purposes, defined the word. The root word is

NAT-

from the Latin NATus, a word that indicates the condition of being born. There are two suffixes added to the word, of which the first creates a noun

$$\text{NAT-ION} \qquad \text{(NA-TION)}$$

while the second transforms the noun into an adjective concept. The same is obviously true for the compounded adjective,

$$\text{VOCA-TION-AL}$$

given earlier. This, again, is not a triplet adjective, but a root with two suffixes.

[15]Structurally the word is a kind of double triplet, a triplet adjective whose root word is itself a triplet. Of course, de-NOMIN-ation is not really a triplet; the suffix -ATION is itself a composite of two suffixes, -ATE and -ION.

[16]All this reminds us of the paradigm concept words,

$$\text{AP-PEASE} \qquad \text{COM-PUTE}$$

which we analyzed earlier. From each of these, one noun concept could be formed to nominalize the action

$$\text{AP-PEASE-MENT} \qquad \text{COM-PUT(E)-ATION}$$

and another to denote the person or device that performs it:

$$\text{AP-PEAS(E)-ER} \qquad \text{COM-PUT(E)-ER}$$

The parallelism is quite striking.

[17]I shall in general use the simpler forms -ATION ($=\bar{a}shn$) and -ATOR ($=\bar{a}\text{-}tor$).

[18]HEART and HEAD are old Anglo-Saxon words; the EA in their spelling might be baffling. CLEAR is a newer French word, and the EA in CLEAR (one can be sure) will always be regularly pronounced. There is some rationale even in the irregularities.

CHAPTER SEVEN

*The Medieval Battle of "Realists" vs. "Nominalists" —
The Conceptualization of Everyday Language: Super-
structure Words in the Vernacular — The Fallacies of
Sight Reading, Speed Reading, Instantaneous Reading —
Reading Is Scanning*

The compounded triplet RE-FRESH-MENT is one of my favorite
paradigms for teaching purposes. The root word

FRESH

is an adjective, from which a verb concept

RE-FRESH

and finally a noun concept

RE-FRESH-MENT

are formed. A root word like FRESH offers no great phonic problems
and as for "meaning" hardly needs an explanation. It has the grammatical standing of an adjective. We can say that fruit is FRESH or
that a child is FRESH. The prefix RE- changes this adjective into a
concept verb: Water is FRESH, it RE-FRESHES, it is RE-FRESH-
ING. Add the suffix -MENT, and you again change a verb concept
into a noun concept:

RE-FRESH-MENT

I hope that this particular and rather simple example will offer
us the means to clarify another, different, and possibly even more

significant aspect of the gradual conceptualization of language. It is an example that even a pupil in elementary school will understand, a word he should easily learn to analyze into components, decode, and read!

Early in his life a child becomes familiar with such things as

APPLES   PEARS
COKE   PEPSI

It is not too long before he understands what is meant by

FRUIT   DRINKS

and the questions that immediately intrude themselves on us are: do words like FRUIT cover concepts or are they still names of things? Have we, by teaching the child to generalize from APPLE to FRUIT, taken him a step toward conceptual thinking? And if, as I said earlier using the word APPLE as paradigm, the names of things cannot be modulated then a further problem arises: can words like FRUIT be modulated; can any kind of new longer words be made out of them to cover more abstract notions or ideas?

To answer these questions is not easy, and students of semantics have been thinking about them for centuries. In fact, the great philosophical battle of medieval scholars, of the so-called "realists" vs. the so-called "nominalists," was fought over this very issue. To put it into simple terms: does such a thing as FRUIT exist as "reality" (in the sense, at any rate, in which medieval Platonic philosophy defined "reality"), or is it only the "name" of something we have abstracted from APPLES and PEARS?[1] Does it exist only in "the mind?"

Medieval philosophers would have called APPLE a "particular," and FRUIT a "universal," and what intrigued them was to what extent "universals" could be considered as being "real." The nominalists tended to question their reality. "Universals," they contended, existed only in the mind.

Of course Abelard, the great nominalist, would never have thought of considering examples as lowly as APPLES and PEARS vs. FRUIT. His much more lofty paradigm was

SOCRATES and PLATO = two "particulars" = real beings
vs.
MAN = a "universal" = a concept[2]

The genius of the language has, so it seems, sided with the "nominalists," at least as far as words like FRUIT are concerned. We cannot add any prefix or suffix to

APPLE

We cannot change its grammatical standing. It is not a concept. But we can turn FRUIT into

FRUITFUL   FRUITION

Moreover, FRUIT is a Latin-derived word, as concept words usually are,[3] whereas APPLE is Germanic. And, most significantly, FRUIT does not name a *thing* as a *Ding-an-sich* but rather in terms of its relationship to us. FRUI is Latin and means *to enjoy;* FRUCTUS means something to be *enjoyed* or *useful;* hence, *edible;* hence, a *produce.* FRUIT is the classical example for naming a thing in terms of its usefulness to us. Still, the word FRUIT looks like a simple root word. We can easily forget its derivation and treat it as the name of a thing. We eat an APPLE; we eat FRUIT. Only when he can quasi-universalize FRUIT, SWEETS, DRINKS, etc., into

REFRESHMENTS

can we say that a child's mind is ready for the great leap toward abstraction and concept formation, the great leap which a restriction of the teaching vocabulary to look-and-say words cannot help but postpone.[4]

Words like

AP-PEASE-MENT

(my paradigm) continue as vocal symbols of conceptual acts even in the nominalized form. They are not easy words for a youngster to understand. There was a reason why I started with this particular type, admittedly a rather difficult example: I thought I should first emphasize the phonic problem. Only secondarily did I turn toward the grammatical aspects of the procedure of forming new, more complex words, especially of changing verb concepts into noun concepts. Subsequently I referred to a less abstract and much more common aspect of noun concept formation in connection with the word

COM-PUT(E)-ER

And now here we have our new paradigm,

RE-FRESH-MENT

These words do not continue as symbols of conceptual acts in the guise of grammatical nouns. They are essentially *names of things*, but with a proviso. More and more the logic of the language will admit these types of words as genuine nouns, as names of things, though as names of things *in terms of their usage*, as names of things *in terms of their relation to us*.[5] This will certainly not be the case with my paradigm "particular,"

APPLE

An APPLE can exist in its Platonic "reality" even without a "mind" thinking of it. I am not quite sure about FRUIT. Neither were the medieval scholars. (Hence their arguments.) And I am even less sure about DRINK (especially the plural form, DRINKS), which is primarily a verb and only recently became, and I think only in American usage, transmuted into a noun, a name of things that are good for a certain thing. As far as our paradigm, RE-FRESH-MENT, is concerned, the word would certainly not exist without a "mind" thinking in terms of concepts. Still, the word is not, for us, a "universal," and the logic of the language puts it, especially its plural form RE-FRESH-MENTS, straight into the category of things: you can serve RE-FRESH-MENTS at a party, and will be just as little cognizant of the realist vs. nominalist dilemma as you might be facing the term FRUIT.[5]

Seemingly, the distinction between "particulars" and "universals" is a fluid one. The words I use may be concept-derived but, when I complain to the SUPER because my A-PART-MENT is cold or my RE-FRIGER-ATOR is leaking, then I am thinking about "real" things, "particulars," regardless of what Abelard or Occam would have said had they ever been faced with these terms.
The triplet noun

RE-FRESH-MENT

is an especially good and simple nontechnical introductory example with which to demonstrate to students quite early in their career how, with the gradual conceptualization of language, we start to name things in terms of usage, of purpose, in terms of relation to us. Actually, it is our technical civilization that has greatly contributed to the evolvement of such words. The names that most readily come to mind in this connection are

AUTO-MOBILE
AIR-PLANE (FLUG-ZEUG, flying machine, in German)
COM-PUT(E)-ER

The first is a hybrid compound of Greek and Latin that tells what it does. The second is a compound of two Latin words much less descriptive than the German equivalent. The third is a triplet noun, a derived word, the typical technical noun concept; the root word is assimilated Latin and the ending is one of several suffixes that turn a verb concept into a noun, a noun that *names a device in terms of what it does.*

In present-day English there is no dearth of words of this type. Most of them are long words, many of them (not all!) are Latin or Greek superstructure words, most of them are easily spotted by endings like

-ER   -OR   -TOR   -ATOR

Any urban American boy from almost any socioeconomic or literacy level will recognize such words when spoken. Here are some examples:

HEAT-ER	TRAN(S)-SIST-OR	AC-CUMUL-ATOR
TRANS-FORM-ER	RE-ACT-OR	AC-CELER-ATOR
DISH-WASH-ER	SE-LECT-OR	E-LEV-ATOR
AIR-CONDITION-ER[6]		IN-CINER-ATOR
LAWNMOW-ER		RE-FRIGER-ATOR[7]

Most of the words ending in -ER, most of the examples in the first cluster, belong in a special group of device names. They are usually not Latin-derived; they have no prefixes, and they are compounds of noun and verb, like DISH-WASH-ER (it WASHes DISHes), or of verb and adverb, like LOUD-SPEAK-ER (it SPEAKS LOUDly). Some stand on their own feet, like HEAT-ER. Only exceptionally do they follow the classic triplet pattern, as in COM-PUT(E)-ER or TRANS-FORM-ER, in which case they are Latin derived.

As for the words in the third cluster of these examples, we might say that, next to our fully analyzed paradigm

AP-PEASE-MENT

with its "twin"

AP-PEAS(E)-ER

they represent the most common and most important contingent of derived nouns. They also derive from concept verbs and usually come in "twins." For an example, see page 116 in the previous chapter. Here are a few more "twins" of derived nouns:

DECOR-AT(E)-ION	DECOR-AT(E)-OR
E-DUC-AT(E)-ION	E-DUC-AT(E)-OR
IN-CINER-AT(E)-ION	IN-CINER-AT(E)-OR

They are nouns formed by subsuffixes from the respective verb concepts

DECOR-ATE   E-DUC-ATE   IN-CINER-ATE

which in turn were derived with the suffix -ATE from roots not in general use. In the first example the root stands naked; in the other two it carries a "prefix."

With the subsuffix -ION, our paradigms furnish the nominalized form of some act. (The relation between suffix and subsuffix is so intimate that in the spoken language they have become a single syllable. What is three syllables, A-TI-O, in Latin, becomes $\bar{a}shn$ in spoken English.) With the subsiffix -OR they specify the device that does it.

Such words exist by the hundreds. Many have become parts of the vernacular. They are all Latin derived. (I cannot think of any exception.) They are superstructure words, and they offer no spelling problems.[8]

As our thinking and speaking become more and more conceptualized, compounded words become, by sheer bulk, dominant in the language not only of the literate but to a certain extent even of the culturally deprived. They certainly become part of the juvenile vocabulary. Not every student will be ready to deal with an admittedly rather complex concept like

AP-PEASE-MENT

but many will understand what

RE-FRESH-MENTS

are, and at least city boys will know what an

IN-CINER-ATOR

is. It is the teacher's job to decide what kinds of complex words to introduce into the taught material. What I must emphasize, however repetitious I may sound, is that there is never any need to learn these words "by heart" or to recognize them "by sight." Scores of these words have the same structure. The problem is to find out, spell out, sound out the root word. The number of prefixes and suffixes is limited. Their sound (and form) can easily be memorized. But even that is unnecessary. They all respond to a simple phonic key. And even their specific role as meaning modifier can easily be learned. (As we just saw in the case of words ending with, say, the suffix

-ATOR

they all name either persons or mechanical devices in terms of what they do.)

There is another aspect of concept word formation still to be considered. Hand in hand with the trend toward the "realization" of words that in their verb form signify conceptual acts (an ELEVATOR elevates, a GOVERNOR governs) goes the opposite trend: the *"sur-réalisation"*[9] of words originally meant to be "real." Basic words, truly basic words, more and more often become conceptualized by the device of changing their grammatical standing. Of course, the borderline between what is concept and what is not is, to quite an extent, artificial, but by now it has also become very fluid. Take the following examples:

I HAND him a GIFT.
I HOUSE a GUEST in my HOME.
I BOOK a PASSAGE.
I am HEAD-ing in the RIGHT DI-REC(T)-TION.
I am HEAD-ing a DE-PART-MENT.
I am the HEAD of a DE-PART-MENT.

The nouns HAND, HOUSE, BOOK, HEAD are non-concept nouns here conceptualized into verbs (except for the word HEAD in the last sentence), while GIFT, GUEST, HOME, RIGHT are concept words *ab ovo*, however basic and Anglo-Saxon their look or sound. What I hand out is "in itself," in its Kantian self, money, liquor, food,[10] candy, cigarettes, or whatnot; it is the interpersonal relationship that makes it a GIFT. It also is the interpersonal relationship that makes a particular person called JOHN DOE a GUEST; and it is the same relationship that makes my house not his HOME. The word PASS-AGE is, of course, a noun concept derived from a verb PASS by adding the noun-forming French-derived suffix -AGE. That RIGHT, DI-REC(T)-TION, DE-PART-MENT are concept words needs no elaboration.

I must add one more thought. At the present stage of American linguistic civilization there are many more good middle-class people who send out

ANNOUNCEMENTS

than people who would bother with the Latin roots of such concept nouns. And there will be people even in the lowest social or literacy stratum complaining about the broken-down RE-FRIGER-ATOR or E-LEV-ATOR, or other

AP-PLI-ANCE

in their

A-PART-MENT

(not DE-PART-MENT, not COM-PART-MENT), and never bothering about what these words actually signify.

This, obviously, is the saddest comment I can make about a system of education that eliminates Greek and Latin from the curriculum while our vocabulary becomes more and more saturated with Greek and Latin. Our more and more conceptualized thinking is utterly unimaginable without a Latin and Greek linguistic super-structure.[11] Even some terrible American neologisms (the British would never commit such lapses of taste), such as

SUPER

for the man who removes the garbage and

LAUNDRO-MAT[12]

for a business which provides washing machines for public use are derivatives from Latin or Greek in which there is at least some concept, however hidden. The liberal German philosopher, Count Keyserling, once decried our civilization as a civilization of automobilists: we all drive cars and don't care to know what is under the hood. More and more we use words and don't know what they mean.

I find the idea quite absurd that a child's reading vocabulary should be restricted to nonconcept words and those few concept words his brain has already covered, but mostly to nonconcept words. New words crop up in our lives all the time. At first we may not know what they are all about. But from the first, a child's mind should be prepared for the idea that only by meeting new and not-yet-known words through reading, will he achieve new insights into an expanding, exciting, interesting world, the world of the grown-ups. The only way to learn to read is by "attacking" words from the very beginning. The tool of the attack is phonic analysis and, in the case of long or longer words, structure analysis.

As far as new words which have not yet been met are concerned, they need not be concept words. A great many of our urban or suburban children don't know at age seven what the words

MARE   COLT   FOAL   STEED

mean; all they know is the word

HORSE

Certainly this is no reason not to know how to read those words, as our "meaning" protagonists must deduce. Take the first of these words. It belongs in a cluster

BARE   CARE   DARE
FARE   HARE   SHARE

which a child at age seven *must* know how to phonemicize, regardless of meaning or understanding, if he has been taught the rule of the silent E and the rule of the modifying R and the digraph SH. The student might not know the meaning of some other words in the cluster. But that is irrelevant. By the time he first meets with any of these words he should know how to pronounce it when he sees it, how to spell it when he writes it.

In the first two years of schooling a child must develop a technique (a "code") by which to do the translation from written to sounded words all through his reading life. This is our way of learning in our present civilization. He cannot afford to have his time wasted. I discover through technical educational publications that some 60 percent of the time a teacher is supposed to teach reading is actually spent in her reading aloud, telling stories, making the lesson "meaningful," "enlarging the children's horizon of experience," etc. It is my considered opinion that this is wasting much of the children's time. They should be given the tools of reading; they should be taught the technique of "de-coding" seriously and systematically without diversion by entertainment. Of course, their horizons should be enlarged by the teacher's reading to them from the Bible, the classics, the masterpieces of literature, and from books on science and history — material which they cannot yet read by themselves. But whether they read or have read to them the uninteresting stories computerized by experts is truly irrelevant. These pieces cannot supply the tools for reading. (Teaching reading calls for clusters of words for practice, clusters of words arranged according to phonic principles, not repetition of words for visual memorizing.) Nor do they enlarge our children's "horizon." (Most of them repeat words and concepts a child already knows.) And their esthetic value is nil.

In the little two-room school which I attended the reading material consisted of poems, fables, histories. Much of the time was taken up by the repeated reading aloud of the same piece. We did the reading, not the teacher. The better students started. Some of the children were poorer readers, coming as they did from less-educated families. After they had heard the same story or poem repeatedly they too did quite well. In any event, reading aloud was a must. Reading aloud in the first school grades is a must, even if it is only a temporary affair.

As one gains more and more experience in reading, the translation of seen words into sounded words becomes practically subconscious (but never eliminated!) and reading aloud, even "lip" reading become an impediment to speed. At the same time the shape, the timeless shape (the *Gestalt,* if you wish), of the written or printed word may acquire meaning beyond what is indicated by the sound. To note the *difference* between

KNIGHT   NIGHT

becomes truly and purely a visual affair. One "looks" and really "sees" the meaning difference via the visual difference. But the time element still remains major and the *Gestalt* element, though present, still remains secondary. As mentioned earlier, both KNIGHT and NIGHT must still be scanned from left to right and the initial N (=/n/) is still read, visually as well as auditorily, *before* the vowel and this *before* the T (= /t/). As far as their sound is concerned, the two words are identical. Still, supported by context we shall hardly ever confuse their meaning if we hear them. The *Gestalt* element does of course help when we see the words in print, and it also adds to the esthetics of English spelling. (I would hate to see KNIGHT spelled NITE or NYT.) But it is certainly not essential.

Reading aloud and writing, let me repeat, are the foundations of sound reading habits. They both help to establish scanning as the time parameter of reading.

Even if our subjective experience tells us that we see the word

G-O-D

"all at once," as a unit in timelessness, the difference between

G-O-D   D-O-G

is still a difference in time. Even if the difference were but a thousandth of a second, we still read the G in G-O-D *visually as much as auditorily* before we read the D. That we take in whole word pictures "all at once" is just not so. This mistaken idea came from the discovery that our eyes stand still for a fraction of a second while we read a substantial portion of a line of print, at first a letter or two as children, later several words, perhaps several lines. *It all happens while the eyes stand still.* Our eyes move over the printed line in so-called saccades, in quick jerks, which on the average take no more than 2/100 of a second (Woodworth, 1938), and *during the individual saccades we are letter-blind.*[13] There is ample time during what the ophthalmograph (an instrument that registers eye movements) describes as the fixation pause *between saccades* to scan over a directionalized sequence of letters visible during this pause, and *only* during this pause, to scan from left to right if the text consists of Latin letters, or from right to left if it is in Hebrew.

Scanning, in my very strict definition, means the directionalized movement of attention across a group of letters or words *with the eyes immobile at the same time.* What the eyes can take in by scanning during the fixation pause is what essentially determines the speed of reading; not the speed of the saccade, which is unchange-able, not the length of the pause, which over a lifetime changes little.

Some people read rapidly, others slowly, but the time element is never negligible.

PAT LOVES TOM

TOM LOVES PAT

are two different statements and whether one hears them or reads them, it is the time element, a sequence element that decides the meaning. We might see the whole of the first sentence in one fixation pause. (Should we rather call it "reading pause" since we do all our reading during this pause?) But we still "read" PAT first, TOM later, within the time span of that *one* "pause."

The question of what is meant by the term "simultaneous" needs to be looked into at this junction. Our brain is obviously better than our mind. For our conscious experience *a time shorter than about 1/50 or 1/30 of a second does not exist.* Anything that happens within the confines of this "elementary moment"[14] appears "simultane-ous" to us. If two electric lights are turned on, each for say 1/1000 of a second, but the second light is turned on 1/100 of a second later than the first, then, *to our subjective experience*, the two light flashes are "simultaneous." We see two lights in two different places *at the same time.* The so-called veridicial value of the information delivered by our sensorium is obviously limited. But that does not mean that the two visual proc-esses *are* "simultaneous." If two such stimuli hit the same retinal area (if the *same* light is turned on twice in quick succession), then the second stimulus might actually interfere with the visual effectiveness of the first. If the second of the two lights is turned on more than 1/5 of a second after the first, we see the "real" sequence of events: one light on and off, followed by *another* light in *another* place on and off. *Two visual stimulus events need to be spearated by about 1/5 of a second to be experienced as two independent sensory events, each possessing its own locus in space and its own moment in time.*

If the second light follows the first light by more than about 1/30 of a second but less than about 1/5 of a second (and if the two look fairly similar and are reasonably close to each other), then we have a strange experience of movement, an illusion: the first light seems to move into the place of the second. We don't see two lights in two places; we don't see what is "real." We see *one* light, moving. This famous so-called phi phenomenon, analyzed by Wertheimer (1912), is the basis of our ability to see a movie the way we do. As everybody now knows, a movie projector presents 24 frames (each repeated once) each second. This makes the pictures appear to be continuous and in motion. In reality, it is consecutive still pictures the brain receives. We just cannot see 48 events or even 24 events per second as independent events.[15]

The critical time span for independent visual experiences is around 1/5 of a second. This is about the length of time our gaze will "rest" on a sequence of letters or words in a fixation pause. There is little variation. It is a little longer, about 1/4 of a second (250 milliseconds), for an average college student (Buswell, 1922). It is a little shorter, perhaps 1/6 of a second (160 milliseconds), for a fast reader, just enough to avoid confluence, the seeing of motion, the phi. It is what we are able to "scan over" during this 1/6 to 1/4 of a second, the duration of a fixation pause, that actually determines our speed of reading. It is its immeasurableness in subjective terms that gives this scanning procedure a sense of simultaneousness. Nevertheless we "scan"; we do not "look." As I said, in the sentence

PAT LOVES TOM

we read PAT *before* we get to TOM. The sentence can all easily be covered during one "pause." We don't need to fixate each letter, each word. If we can "cram"

PAT LOVES TOM DEARLY   (1)

or even

PAT LOVES TOM PASSIONATELY   (2)

into one pause we are doing still better. Strangely, sentence 2 requires hardly any more time than sentence 1, while

PAT LOVES HER GRAY CAT TOM   (3)

takes considerably longer to read though, counting the letters and the space between words, sentence 2 and 3 are exactly the same length. As Woodworth (1938) states: "Presumably, a familiar long word, being a coherent whole, requires less scrutiny than an equal space fitted with short words." And then comes the crowding of contours and the lack of it (which will be discussed in Chapter Nine); this leaves the two ends of even relatively long conglomerations of letters relatively recognizable although their images fall onto retinal loci considerably removed from the area of best vision.

But let me repeat: The fact that we can cover several words "at a glance," meaning during one fixation pause, does not mean that we "look and see" all these words as *Gestalten*, as patterns, simultaneously. Those 160 to 250 milliseconds leave ample time for attention to proceed, for scanning, for scanning *without moving* the eyes. (Moving them would only blur the retinal images.) Not only the words, but also the letters within words are taken in by scanning, in a definite sequence that involves time. Even in the short word

GOD

we see and perceive the letter G *before* we see and perceive the letter D, conditioned as we are, conditioned if we are, to write and read from left to right.

With a bow to the "meaning" school, we should add here that the reading language of the cultured adult is replete with words he will most likely never hear, only see. Many of the examples given earlier are that kind of word. Our spoken language is amazingly restricted. We have a home vocabulary (these are the words relied upon by the "meaning" school of teaching); we have a vocabulary for our professional life; and a vocabulary for our social contacts. (I found it requires no more than about fifty words or phrases in an otherwise strange language to conduct a meaningful conversation with a patient during an eye examination.) All these words are constantly repeated. But our intellectual interests bring us in contact in reading with thousands of words we may never have a chance to pronounce. "Why, then, in their case bother with phonics?" seems a justified question. Perhaps in the long run "phonics" is not even the right term for the teaching technique outlined here. It is in fact rather a technique of keys, a technique for attacking words with clues, a "de-coding," and, in contradistinction to the look-and-say method, an analytic rather than an associative technique or approach. And as this and the previous chapter reveal, "de-coding for sound" is only part of the teaching and learning business. With the continued conceptualization of the language, even for those of elementary school age, "de-coding of structure" becomes an integral part of the reading process, of the process a teacher must teach and a student must learn.

There is one more comparative linguistic item to be considered before one passes judgment on the merits and demerits of the look-and-say method. There must be some reason why it was initiated in an English-speaking country. There is some justification for the method. First of all, English has an inordinately large number of homophones, and this favors visual separation according to meaning (KNIGHT/NIGHT, PIECE/ PEACE). Even more: the simplicity of English grammar allows relative stability of words. Hungarian (expressing grammatical relations with the help of affixes, often multiple) stands at the opposite pole in this respect. Thus, the visual image of a great many English words hardly changes and this allows them to be memorized; they are in fact memorized inadvertently. KNIGHT can become

KNIGHTS   KNIGHT'S

(KNIGHT-LY   KNIGHT-HOOD)

A word like LOVE, which is both a noun and a verb, hardly sports more forms than one can count on the fingers of one hand:

LOVES   LOVE'S   LOVED

LOVING   LOVER

(BE-LOVED   UN-LOVED)

are about all I can think of. All grammatical problems involve auxiliaries. In contradis- tinction, the visual image of Hungarian words constantly changes. "I LOVE you" and "He fell in LOVE with her" are whole sentences in English with the word LOVE pre- senting itself as an unchanged visual image. In Hungarian, each of these sentences presents itself as a single word (the first one three and the second five syllables long), with the base word visually hidden among prefixes and suffixes needed to modify the base word's meaning in the appropriate manner. A look-and-say technique for teaching Hungarian children to read is almost unthinkable.

NOTES

[1]On page 117, I used the noun INSTRUMENT in another context. We could ask the same question relating to this word: does such a thing as an instrument exist as a "reality?" Or is the word merely a "name" abstracted from "violins" and "trom- bones?"

[2]The battle of the "realists," the establishment, the hierarchy, against "nominal- ist" heresy was not, to be sure, merely a battle over the nature of nouns, even a noun like MAN. Much deeper issues were involved. What those like St. Bernard were against was nominalist (we would call it liberal) speculation about such items of faith as the "reality" of the Trinity — one of the great, great issues in medieval thought.

[3]Significantly, FRUIT comes from the Latin FRUI for "enjoy," "making use of." The Latin word describes a thing in terms of its usefulness to us. Still, FRUIT has be- come part of the basic language. It is by now *almost* a name of things. How truly it has become a basic word is revealed by the fact that in German the Latin word FRUCTUS has taken up the form

FRUCHT

with (what I half-jokingly call) the "Teutonc" ending-CHT. But that it is a concept word, nevertheless, is shown by such a derived form as

be-FRUCHT-en = to fertilize

a verb concept for whose meaning English needed a long superstructure word stemming from the Latin FERre (to bear).

[4]"*Ratio est oratio*," said the great English philosopher, Thomas Hobbes: "Thought is essentially the same as speech." Thus, when concept words are withheld, conceptual thinking is retarded.

[5]In the examples given earlier,

AP-PEAS-ER   VOT-ER   JUDGE   etc.

we found a related tendency: to name a person in terms of what he does.

[6]AIR-CONDITION-ER is composed of two nouns of which the second is itself a compounded Latin-derived noun.

[7]The suffixes will sometimes signify a person rather than a device, as in

WAIT-ER	GOVERN-OR	JANI-TOR
AN-NOUNC(E)-ER	SENAT(E)-OR	TU-TOR
	TRANS-LAT(E)-OR	DECOR-ATOR

Sometimes, as in the case of CONDUCT-OR, the word can signify either a person or a thing. The suffix -AR, as in RE-GIST(E)R-AR, and the suffix -YER, as in LAW-YER, SAW-YER, refer only to people.

[8]There are, of course, no clear-cut categories. In our examples AD-MIR-ATION and DE-CLAR-ATION the theoretical in-between verb forms AD-MIR-ATE and DE-CLAR-ATE have withered away as unnecessary and the "twin" AD-MIR-ATOR never developed.

[9]I apologize for the expression, but the French word *surréal* has specific connotations, having to do with the manipulation of reality, whereas the word "surrealistic" has by now become part of our vernacular.

[10]The choice of the example FOOD seems inappropriate though it was chosen with a purpose. Actually FOOD is a concept word defining variegated items in terms of their use to us. The example shows how difficult it is to separate nouns (= names of things) into what Abelard would have considered names of "real" things and other names. When APPLE becomes FRUIT, and FRUIT becomes FOOD, and FOOD becomes GIFT we are several times removed from Abelard's "reality."

[11]I want to mention as an aside that the use of Latin and Greek superstructure words offers the only possibility for that international concept language toward which we are steering so hopefully and so inexorably. H-A-T means, as we saw, different things in English and German but

TRANSISTOR RADIO

means the same thing in both languages, even if the English pronounce the A in radio as /ā/. And the Germans would do well to stop calling OXYGEN *Sauerstoff* when the word OXYGEN is used all over the world.

It is, by the way, through the wholehearted acceptance of these Latin-derived words that (with some generous though inadvertent help from the French) English is rapidly becoming the international tongue. The Germans made the wrong move toward such ambition. They use the word *Erzieher* for our EDUCATOR and the word *gebildet* for our EDUCATED, beautiful words that with their deeper meanings and exquisite connotations will continue to be cherished by all who love and appreciate the German language — evey by those who are not too enthusiastic about its use of *Sauerstoff* for OXYGEN, *Fernsprecher* for TELEPHONE, or *Augenheilkunde* for OPHTHALMOLOGY. We might, half in earnest, also add that through the wholehearted acceptance of all these Latin words (they now make up a large part of the English vernacular) English is more and more becoming a Romance tongue, and that the conquests of Caesar and the papacy of Rome could not achieve what English is now accomplishing: it is through English that Latin is now conquering the world.

Of course, the magnificent simplicity of English grammar also helps. (Who wants to bother with an international language which has three genders or seven cases? Or a language with its own alphabet?) The whole process could be accelerated if only textbooks for foreigners did not continue with such false and deplorable statements as that English spelling is "difficult," "irregular," "appalling," and "unlearnable."

As far as the role of Greek is concerned, that is a different story. The internationally accepted Greek-origin scientific terms are not meant to become part of the vernacular. They are often unnecessarily abstruse. Without looking it up in a dictionary who knows what

PLEISTOCENE

stands for? However, more and more people know by now what

CHROMOSOME

means, and

HELICOPTER

has become a vernacular word.

[12]To me, this word is a kind of eyesore. The semiliterate copywriter who invented it obviously did not know that in

AUTO-MAT

it is the first half of the word, and not the second half, that suggests "do-it-yourself."

For some reason, I have no bad feelings about BUS and AUTOBUS, used in lieu of "omnibus" and "automobile omnibus." Although the word BUS is actually meaningless, I find it not without charm as an abbreviation.

[13]We don't "register" details of optical images *while* they are sliding across the retina.

[14]See the exposition on biological time by Von Uexküll and Kriszat (1924), one of the most charming biological-philosophical essays I have ever read.

[15]I am told that the older movie projector presented each frame once. This often caused pictures to flicker. The flickering can be helped by running the reel faster, and it is this that gives strangeness to old movies: everybody is constantly on the run, and the wheels of trains often appear to be running backward.

CHAPTER EIGHT

*On the Directedness of Written Letters and Written (or
Printed) Words — Historical Notes on the Development of
Some Hebrew and Latin Letters — Why Will Poor Readers
Confuse p and q? — Why Will Poor Readers Read W-A-S
for S-A-W or G-R-I-L for G-I-R-L?*

Lefthanded Sumerians or Persians, had such people ever been in the
majority, would certainly have started their cuneiforms on the right
side of their clay tablets. This would have been the way to avoid
smudging. And a tribe of Greeks with a lefthanded majority, had one
ever existed, would have established a system of writing that would
look like mirror writing to us. *Neither would have introduced what
we might call the Semitic writing idiom.* It is amazing that even experts on writing often do not realize the basic difference. Hebrew
letters, written from right to left, are still written by the right hand.
The strokes that constitute them are righthanded strokes. Hebrew
writing is not mirror writing even though the static picture of individual Hebrew letters sometimes suggests this. It certainly is not
lefthanded writing.[1]

To clarify this point I shall try to show, through a few letter sam-
ples, that individual written letters possess what I like to call an
intrinsically directional character, that this character is determined
by the fact that we use the right hand, and that this character is lost
or hidden in most of our printed letters. I believe that only by writing,
and not by reading, can one become truly cognizant of this intrinsically directional character of letters, printed letters included. In
addition to all this analysis I have a clinical purpose in mind. I hope
to bring home the point that even when we let an apparently left-

140

handed child write with the left hand we have not solved all his problems. What we are, by necessity, forcing this child to do is write
righthanded characters with the wrong hand — the left. I hope that
my analysis of this intrinsic directional character of written letters will be found relevant to the problem of writing in general and to
the problem of reading difficulties in particular. I shall start with
aleph or A, the first letter of most of the alphabets.

The original ideogram,[2] representing an ox, called aleph in
Hebrew, must have looked like

$$\aleph \quad \text{or} \quad \text{\Large \texttt{ʊ}}$$

At one point in the development of Semitic writing (it developed
along several almost independent lines), the picture, the ideogram,
became the symbol of a sound, of a consonant. It is the first sound
picture in a great many alphabets. This being so, it is strange that
this sound value is now practically forgotten. (In transliteration linguists simply mark the presence of the letter with an apostrophe
/'/. For practical purposes, all this matters little. At the moment, we
are more interested in the letter than in its sound.

At some time during the history of its use as a sound symbol the
direction of the aleph character was changed by 90 degrees. This 90-
degree turn of what originally was a picture, an ideogram, is not at all
unknown in the developmental course of ancient scripts. We also
encounter it in the history of the cuneiform script (Diringer, 1962).
It has to do with the fact that the Near-Eastern scribes finally opted
for writing along horizontal, instead of vertical lines, and they found it
easier to make imprints or brush strokes horizontally rather than vertically. Thus, the Hebrews, writing from right to left, finally transformed the ideogram for ox into their letter aleph[3]:

$$\infty = \text{IC} = \underset{2 \ 1}{\text{↓G}} \ \leftarrow$$

(with the ideogram turned 90 degrees toward the left), and the Greco-
Romans, writing from left to right, into

$$\alpha \, (= \ \text{ᄃ}) = \text{CL} = \underset{1 \ 2}{\rightarrow\text{G G}} = a$$

(with the ideogram turned the other way).[4] Both symbols are meant to
be written with the right hand, both are cursive forms, i.e., forms to
be written, not printed, and they are not mirror images of each other
in terms of writing kinetics. Both the Hebrew aleph and the Latin a

are written in two steps (even if in cursive Latin the pen is not necessarily lifted between them), and the first stroke, the semicircle
(marked by the number 1), is written in the same direction (the direction indicated by an arrow head). The second stroke, the vertical
(marked by the number 2), follows the semicircle — in Hebrew on the
left side, in Latin on the right, because (as the horizontal arrows
indicate) the gaze of the Hebrew scans toward the left, and that of
the Latin toward the right. A lefthander, intent on writing what to us
is the mirror image of the cursive Latin a would present us with the
pattern

$$\text{ⅉ} = \text{ⅉ}\underset{2}{}\underset{1}{} \leftarrow$$

with a letter that is far from being identical with the Hebrew aleph.
Hebrew writing is righthanded writing from right to left; it is not
mirror writing.

Let me use the letters T and the Y as further paradigms, two
symmetrical capital letters, not too different from each other in the
printed capital letter form. A child reared on "writing first" will feel
the direction of the line that crosses the T in the muscles of his hand.
Written t's

$$\boldsymbol{t}, \boldsymbol{\mathcal{T}}, \boldsymbol{\mathcal{T}} = \quad \rightarrow \underset{1}{\boldsymbol{t}}^{2} \text{ or } \underset{2}{\boldsymbol{\mathcal{T}}}^{1} \text{ or } \underset{1}{\boldsymbol{\mathcal{T}}}^{2}$$

are not symmetrical and carry the direction left to right in every detail
of their structure. So does their cognate, the Hebrew TAV

$$\text{ת} = \underset{2}{}\underset{1}{} \leftarrow$$

which is a no less righthanded letter than either of the written Latin
letters t or T. Especially note the horizontal stroke of the Latin written capital letter. Its direction, left to right, is not subject to choice
whichever stroke is written first.)[5]

The letter Y is also symmetrical as a printed capital. In its written form the letter is made up of two strokes (even if, in cursive writing, the pen is not being lifted):

$$\boldsymbol{y} = \boldsymbol{y} = \rightarrow \overset{1}{\boldsymbol{\mathcal{Y}}}\underset{2}{}$$

There is a definite directional sequence built into this performance
pattern. The stroke on the left (marked by the number 1) is the first of
the two strokes, and this is not subject to choice: both the hand and
the gaze of a righthander run in the direction indicated by the hori-

zontal arrow. Moreover, the direction of each stroke in itself is given
and is not subject to choice. To write

$$\overset{1}{\mathsf{U}}\overset{2}{\mathsf{J}}$$

would be against the flow of the hand and would cause the ink to
splutter, although the final outcome would be correct. To put the
individual strokes on paper in the natural righthanded manner but
in reversed order, thus,

$$\overset{2}{\mathsf{U}}\overset{}{\mathsf{J}}{}_1$$

would also be unnatural. It would be against the direction of gaze.
Besides, neither form permits the second stroke to join the first one,
which is what, after all, gives a *raison d'être* and desirable speed to
cursive writing. Certainly a letter like the written y or Y is rigorously
directionalized; to a reader reared on writing, the memory of the
written letter will always be present even when he looks at the symmetrical letters T or Y in print.

As the next examples I have chosen two symbols each of which
might have been chosen to denote the sound /k/ or /kh/. The word
KOS means "cup" or "chalice" in Hebrew,[6] and the word KAPH
means the palm of the hand as used for drinking. The original ideograms must have been

$$\mathsf{Y} \text{ or } \mathsf{U}$$

a goblet with stem and foot or a half circle. For ease in writing, such
ideograms were in time turned 90 degrees in one direction or the
other. The half-circle, turned left, survives in the Hebrew letter actually called KAPH:

$$\mathsf{D} = \mathsf{D} \leftarrow$$

which, turned toward the right, gives us the third letter of the Latin
alphabet:

$$\mathsf{c} = \rightarrow \mathsf{G}$$

Both the Hebrew and the Latin letter sound like /k/ much of the time
(but not all). In fact, the Latin letter originally must have always
sounded like /k/.

CICERO

the man whom the English and the Italians respectively call

sisero and *chichero*

was by the Latins most likely called

kikero

Talmudic transliteration of Latin words is one good reason to assume this.[7]

The other, and much more interesting form, clearly a goblet turned 90 degrees, appears to have been first written from right to left

$$\exists = \overset{\displaystyle ?}{\underset{2}{}}\overset{\displaystyle /}{\underset{1}{}} \leftarrow$$

by both Semites and Greeks. Since the Greeks, in their practical and rational manner, finally opted for writing from left to right they turned the symbol around to become their kappa, our

$$\kappa = K = \rightarrow \underset{1}{/}\underset{2}{\mathsf{S}}$$

to be written with the left stroke first. As it happens, the two versions *are* mirror images of each other even in a kinetic-kinesthetic sense. I am quite sure that the reason the Greeks so resolutely eliminated their original choice, writing from right to left, was that the kinetics of this writing just doesn't suit the right hand. As can be seen, there is not a single Greek or Latin letter in which a stroke like

$$\textrm{> or ⏎ or 7 or U}$$

would have survived. Ink will splutter if the nib of a quill pen or of a round-hand pen is forced to draw such lines with the right hand. Even the Hebrews tried to eliminate such lines with time while they continued to write from right to left with the right hand.

A good example of this is our letter L. It comes from the Semitic ideogram for the ox goad, lamed. In modern Hebrew print and cursive Hebrew the respective letters look like this:

$$\textrm{ל} \leftarrow \textrm{ and } \textrm{ſ} \leftarrow$$

while the Latin forms are

$$\rightarrow \textrm{4 and } \rightarrow \textrm{ℓ}$$

In both instances the *written* letters are meant to be written by the right hand and the horizontal line runs toward the right in both the

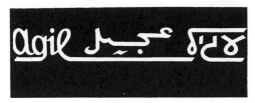

Fig. 2. A Jerusalem shop window: the four letters A-G-I-L in three different cursives. Note the similarity of Latin and Hebrew. The letter G extends downward, the letter L extends upward in both Latin and Hebrew. Note also that the "wings" of both Hebrew letters ﬤ = g and ﬢ = l run toward the right since they were written by the right hand. Note furthermore that, although the writing is cursive, each Hebrew letter is written separately. Note, finally, the letter ﬩ = l at the end of the Arabic word. It is an "inverted" image of the Hebrew.

Hebrew and the Latin. They are certainly not mirror images of each other.[8]

A trilingual sign in a Jerusalem shop window (Fig. 2) shows the difference in the character of the two Semitic scripts, Hebrew and Arabic, although both of them run from right to left. The name of the store is AGIL. In the Hebrew transliteration, on the right, one sees four separate characters. The GIMEL (*G*) and the LAMED (*L*) sport exaggerated horizontal strokes directed from left to right in the technically advantageous direction for a pen in the right hand. Cursive Hebrew letters have to be written separately to make this possible. Hebrew words are not meant to be and cannot easily be written without lifting one's pen, which is one of the great technical handicaps of Hebrew cursive.

The Arabic transliteration of the word, in the center, is executed without lifting the pen, in the true cursive manner, and even those who cannot read the word will recognize the cognate Arabic letter

$$\text{LAM} = \textbf{ʋ} \;\leftarrow$$

at the left end. The letter is written in the original, time-honored, but less practical way — from right to left.

It would be interesting to examine how first the Greeks and then the Romans handled most of the other letters of the Semitic alphabet, but I shall restrict my discussion to the analysis of one more letter example, an example which in a curious way is pertinent to the dyslexia problem. This letter is the Hebrew QOPH. I don't know of any sure ideographic antecedent. (One of the guesses of linguists is that the original meaning of the symbol was "helmet.") It does not really matter. The fact is that in Hebrew, writing from right to left (and, of course, with the right hand), one traces the sound symbol in two steps:

$$QOPH = P = \underset{2}{}\underset{1}{}$$

and arrives at a pattern reminiscent of the Latin letter P (this is an important detail!), while in Latin the same sound symbol, written from left to right, became

$$Q \text{ or } q = \rightarrow \underset{1 \ 2}{}$$

which in all respects, especially that of writing kinetics, *is* a mirror image of the Hebrew character.

The Greeks left the matter at first undecided, writing their KOPPA like

$$\varphi$$

But, practicalists and antitraditionalists as they were, they soon dropped the letter altogether. Having assimilated the K and created a χ, they needed no third sign for a similar sound.

Parenthetically may I add here that nowhere has the greatness of Greek practical and rational thinking revealed itself better than in their creation of an alphabet from the aleph-bet. Unlike the English, the Greeks were no traditionalists. They would drop a letter (e.g., the Hebrew VAV), if it did not cover any Greek sound. They also dropped letters that they felt were duplications, for example, the SADHE, or the QOPH just mentioned. But their epochal contribution was the creation of signs for vowels, missing in Semitic writing. The Greeks simply used some of the (for them) superfluous Semitic consonant characters ALEPH, HÉ, KHET, YAD, and AYYIN and recreated them into alpha, epsilon, éta, iota and omikron.[9] Thus, they created a complete set of letters, the first complete alphabet, the basis of all European alphabets, ours included.

Discarding of letters did, of course, create some problems, and at least one winding story I find fascinating. I shall relate it purely for its entertainment value:

Greek, like Semitic, letters also served as numbers. The VAV, sounding most probably like our /v/, was the sixth letter in the Semitic prototype alphabets and was therefore generally used as a symbol for "six." (Our number 6 is an inverted VAV.) Imagine the confusion of ledgers and of international trade if the Z = ZAYYIN = ZETA, the seventh letter and the sign for "seven" to Greek and Semite, had suddenly become a "six" to the Greeks because the VAV was dropped from their final, official alphabet. It was much simpler to retain the Z as the sign of "seven" (we have still retained it in our number 7) and to create a new number sign, called the DIGAMMA (literally a "double three") to fill in for "six." The Greek numeral for "three" was Γ = GAMMA[10]; the form of the new number was F. It was a kind of redoubling of the Γ. By the strange and devious ways of history, a letter of exactly the same shape, our F, became in the end the sixth letter in the Latin alphabet. The Latins did need a letter for their sound /f/ and to put it in the place of the VAV seemed logical to them, /f/ and /v/ being related consonants. But the Latins also needed a place for a letter of the sound /g/. This sign, the G (a cognate of the Hebrew GIMEL = camel), they put in the seventh position to replace the ZETA for which *they* had no use. Of course, as far as the /g/ was concerned, this was a place of exile: the letter for the sound /g/ occupies third place, GIMEL and GAMMA, respectively, in the original alphabets, and our number 3 still reminds us of this fact. The Latins placed the ambivalent letter C into the third niche of their arrangement, a letter with the main sound value /k/ related to /g/.[11] In the end they discarded the Greek KAPPA for which they had no use and which brings us back to KOPPA and to the Q, a letter that reached the Latin via the Western Greek and the Etruscan alphabets. How the Phoenician and Greek merchants resolved a possible confusion about the numerical values of QOPH and KOPPA I don't exactly know. All I know is that QOPH for Hebres has the number value 100 while SADHE. the preceding character, is 90. The Greeks never bothered with the latter, to them unneeded, letter, and this gave KOPPA the value of 90. In the end, KOPPA was also dropped as a letter: still it remained a numeral (the Greek sign for 90), while for the Semitic merchant QOPH continued to symbolize 100. (I could never figure out, I once remarked jokingly, who, in the end, cheated whom. Was it the Greek who shipped 90 barrels of oil to Semitic Carthage and billed them for 100, or was it the other way around?)

But this is still only the beginning of my q story. Dyslexic children supposedly mix up q's and p's, a favorite item in the strephosymbolia legend. If the teaching is poor, if it does not begin with writing, with the inculcation of kinetic-kinesthetic training, then a q might be confused with a p by a child. After all the two *are* in the same pattern, mirror images of each other, *if* the pattern does not contain the kinesthetics of its origination. But as soon as we are not unmindful of this, of the *inherent vectorial character* even of the printed letters, we shall realize that this is far from being the case. The Latin *is*, as we have noted, the mirror image of the Hebrew

but it is not a mirror image of the Latin

$$p = $$

I might add that the Hebrew

$$QOPH = $$

and the Latin

$$p = $$

are not identical kinetic patterns, are not identical scanning images, however similar their final static images may look. Only the static *Look-Sally-Look* technique of teaching reading before teaching writing can result, as I know it does, in a child's confusing a p and a q.

The point is so essential that I must be repetitious. Let me therefore analyze the letters q and p once more, this time in terms of their assumed origins. As I said earlier, the letter QOPH may have been the representation of a helmet. *One puts the helmet on first and only then pulls down the visor*, whether one is a Hebrew:

a Latin:

or a mirror-writing lefthanded American:

(Such imaginative descriptions help to add a sense of kinetics to teaching writing of the letters!) In the end, the "helmet" drawn by the Hebrew and the lefthander look very much like an ordinary printed Latin p. However, there is a difference.

Let us look at the history of the letter p for a moment. The name comes from the Hebrew word PÉ for mouth (it sounds like the English word PAY). *You have to start with the ideogram of a man* (which, as we shall see, even in Chinese is essentially a vertical line) *before you can indicate his mouth*. Thus, the prototype of the letter p is not unlike the cursive capital letter I learned in school. In Hebrew,[12] this letter finally assumed the form

$$(\cdot 2 \overline{4]} \leftarrow)$$
$$1$$

while in Latin it came to look like

$$\overrightarrow{1} \diagup \underset{2}{\text{?}} (= \;\; \rightarrow\!\!\mathcal{p}, \text{ in cursive})$$

Obviously the vertical line is drawn first in both instances and the curved line follows — in Hebrew on the left, as expected, in Latin on the right, again as expected. Certainly q and p are different kinetic-kinesthetic images. They are not mirror images. In the Latin alphabet both are oriented in the direction left to right. One is still a helmet with a visor (round part first), and the other is a man with a mouth (the up and down line first).

There is no point in continuing such an analysis for the other pairs of letters poor readers allegedly confuse. Still I think we are justified in some generalization. I honestly feel that if a child ever confuses Latin, p and Latin q, b and d, n and u, or m and w, favorite examples given in the dyslexia literature, then this happens only because the teacher failed to teach the child to "see" and "feel" the movement of his own hand in the creation (note the word "creation") of letter symbols for the questionable advantages of seeing static patterns with stated meanings. These classic examples of strepho-symbolia have in reality little to do with confused laterality, with mixed dominance, perceptual immaturity, etc. The trouble is that the child has not been taught that p's and q's, b's and d's, etc., *all have to flow from left to right*. Letters are not static images; timeless *Gestalten*. They are vectors. They are patterns with a time sequence, just as are the whole words as they finally emerge from the sequence of such letters. These repeated statements about brain damage causing a child to mix up p and q or b and d lack, in my estimation, all basis.[13] All that these examples prove is the inadequacy of our teaching techniques. In that little school (two rooms for six grades) which I attended more than sixty years ago, writing letters was taught by the now detested "rote" method. First the children had to fill pages with lines, line elements of letters: lines flowing from lower left to upper right. Only then came letters. I don't remember that in that school in Hungary a child ever had confused letters. For a child imbued with the kinesthetic memory of letters he had learned to write, letters like

$$\rightarrow \text{ p and } \rightarrow \text{ q}$$

are entirely different kinetic images, even in the abstract modern printed form.

Another item frequently repeated in the literature on dyslexia needs to be examined here in some detail. According to the authorities, who seemingly quote this instance from each other, it is typical for the dyslexic child to confuse S-*A*-*W* and W-*A*-*S* because of strephosymbolia. Some authors are so unmindful of the problem they present that they don't even bother telling us if the child to whom this allegedly happened read *saw* instead of *was* or *was* instead of *saw*.[14] We can assume with some assurance that most probably it was the common auxiliary verb *was* with which this (by now legendary) child became familiar at first. We can assume that this child knew his letters. He has learned somehow (details in these reports are never specified) that the first symbol on the left side is pronounced /w/ and that the symbol on the right side is voiced as /z/. He also knew the vowel that connects the two sounds. He has learned furthermore that the symbol on the left side is to be pronounced first. Knowing all this, but no more (no phonics taught, nothing ever said about directedness of letters within word "images"), an intelligent child must become utterly frustrated when confronted with the pattern

S-A-W

because the naturally assumed sound sequence /z/-/a/-/w/ just has no meaning! It speaks for a child's inventiveness and intelligence, not of his affliction with strephosymbolia, that he tries it the other way around and is rewarded by a familiar and meaningful sound sequence! The child will be especially prone to do this if the compulsion to see *vectors* in words, not *patterns*, has not yet been firmly established. Educators tell us that it takes one to two years before the vectorial character of printed symbols and words establishes itself as a reflex of unconditioned fixity. (Why not teach it from the beginning?) Even the brightest child might reverse letters or words in the first year of learning to read, *especially if he is not first taught to write.*

In order to read the three letters

S-A-W

in a manner that gives meaning to the sequence of pronounced sounds, the law of reading letters in sequence has to be partially superseded. The child has to know, first of all, what vowels are. Then he has to know that certain letters or letter combinations act as retroactive modifiers of *preceding* vowels without themselves being pronounced. He also has to know about the silent E, the silent GH, and, what is relevant for the present example, the silent W. How can a child handle a word like S-A-W if he has not been taught to sound letters in sequence *from left to right,* and has not been familiarized with the principles of vowel modification? I am quite confident that a child that has learned the sound value of the letter combination AW through such example clusters as I have described will never read W-A-S for S-A-W.

As my next example of letter reversal in words I shall cite the one quoted by Dr. Virginia Lubkin in her thought-provoking introduction to a symposium on reading disabilities held in 1967 at the New York Academy of Medicine. The word presented was

GIRL

the word read was

gril

Clearly, again the cause of such reversal is lack of familiarity with the rules of retroactive modification rather than strephosymbolia. Just because the word "GIRL" is such a common word, well known *by sound* and *by meaning* to the youngest pupil, it should not be introduced haphazardly into a child's reading vocabulary. It is a difficult word to spell. The letter R in words like

RIM	PRIM
GRIM	PRIME
GRIME	PRINT

does not affect the sound of the letter I because it precedes the vowel. However, in a cluster of words like

FIR   STIR   FIRM   SKIRT   SIR

the I-plus-R form an indissoluble sound sequence with a modified vowel sound. If such words are prematurely presented, before the phonic value of the letter combination IR has been clarified, the student cannot help becoming confused.

Nor is this the whole story. The word G-I-R-L is a real cracker-jack. One could have hardly presented a more difficult word to a child who has not been taught his phonics.

A child trained in phonics should and will know that, in G-U-N and in G-I-N, in G-A-M-E and in G-E-M, in R-A-N-G and in R-A-N-G-E, the letter G does not symbolize the same sound value. The I and the E quasi-modify what we would call the "principal" sound of the letter G. But — and this is what is unusual — G does not have the same sound value in G-I-N as it does in G-I-R-L or G-I-R-D. The only explanation I can give is that the letter I in these two last words does not represent a sound in the I family any longer! Obviously, the peculiar /ûr/ sound of the I-plus-R combination does not modify the sound of G. Indeed, a word like GIRL is a source of utter confusion when presented to a child not versed in phonics. The child will certainly try his best. He will try to turn the pattern of letters into a complex of sounds that has meaning. He will try /j/-/i/-/r/-/l/, he will try /j/-/u/-/r/-/l, both of which make no sense, and then may try once more and (as Lubkin's patient did) choose

$$/g/-/r/-/i/-/l/$$

which at least is an acceptable form of some faintly familiar word. Children hate exceptions. *Children crave law and order.* A word, a sequence of letters, like

G-I-R-L

has no meaning if pronounced as written. It becomes an "irregularly" spelled or an "irregularly" pronounced word, an exercise in frustration. But the same sequence of letters can become just one in a cluster of examples, not an exception, once the new rules have been established in the child's mind, once the child has been familiarized with the rule of the modified G and what we might call the rules (or pranks) of the "modifying R." All of these, let us be frank, are extremely difficult for the poor reader to master. As I said earlier: "It is not easy to learn to spell English; it is not easy to teach English spelling." Still, it has to be done.

What I have just elaborated on at seemingly undue length is not just an insignificant detail. It happens to throw another interesting

light upon the relationship between spoken and written English. If I
stated earlier that a G is made to sound as /j/ by an I that follows, I
did not accurately formulate the rule. It would have been more accurate had I stated that it is the *sounds* usually represented by the
letter I (i.e., the sounds /i/ and /ĭ/) that modify the sound represented
by the letter G. The *unusual sound* /ûr/, which here happens to be
represented by the letter combination I-plus-R, does not modify the
usual sound of the G. This must be so obvious that in the case of
GIRL or GIRD the founding fathers of our spelling did not even
bother with a demodifier. The situation must have looked entirely
different to them in the case of words like

GUILD or GUILT   GUIDE or GUILE

where we seemingly do need a reminder, black on white, *not* to
change the normal sound of the G. In these examples the letter I
symbolizes the basic /i/ or the modified /ī/ sound, and without the
visual reminder, the demodifier, the reader would be inclined to pronounce the G as /j/.

I realize that there are exceptions. Words like

GILD (to cover with gold)   GET   GIVE

must be mentioned. Also the words

GERM   GERMANY

don't follow my reasoning. G sounds like /j/ in these two examples, in spite of the /ûr/
sound that follows. But it is better to have rules and occasional exceptions for which a
cause is not immediately evident than to have a written language in which there are no
rules, only "irregularities," so that every single word has to be looked at, spoken, and
memorized. (As for GILD we have the excuse that it is a homophone of GUILD, while
GET and GIVE are such old words that they escape the rules.)

NOTES

[1]As I noted earlier, a more serious student of script than I am would more often
refer to Semitic, especially Phoenician, writing and from the point of view of historic
development this is certainly more justified. I shall in this discussion generally refer to
Hebrew writing simply because I am more familiar with it.

[2]An ideogram actually represents some state in a long process of development. It is a picture stripped to essentials. The adjective "original" does not fit it too well.

[3]In the diagrams of written letters which follow, numbers will indicate the sequence of strokes and arrowheads the end point (and the direction) of individual strokes, while horizontal arrows will indicate the general direction of the writing, the direction of both hand and gaze.

[4]The Greek alpha must have also been influenced by the Egyptian hieroglyphic

$$\partial\!\!\!\ell \rightarrow \alpha \text{ or A}$$

Originally this letter was the representation of a hawk. It is one of the handsomest letters in the Egyptian alphabet.

[5]In contradistinction, watch a lefthander's cursive t: *he* crosses his t's from right to left even while writing from left to right.

[6]The primary purpose of these examples is to emphasize and illustrate the directionalized character of letters. How much of the details is historically correct matters less. There is no definite proof that, e.g., the letters C and K came into existence in this quite plausible manner. Some authors believe, for instance, that the Greek KAPPA hails from an Egyptian source.

[7] The transliteration of the word

CAESAR

(in Talmudic times the word meant "emperor") starts in Talmudic Hebrew with the letter QOPH the sound of which is never anything but /k/. The Hebrews of that time must have heard the emperor referred to as

kāsar or *kīsahr*

(vowel values are never sure in old Hebrew texts). And, of course, the Germans also speak of their

kīzer

the word beginning with a /k/ sound when pronounced.

[8]This is not strictly true. If one places a mirror parallel to the line of letters, the upright Latin letter

$$\mathsf{L}$$

will look like the Hebrew letter

$$\curvearrowright$$

in the mirror. But this is not what we generally mean by "mirror image." If one wants to transform Leonardo's mirror writing into ordinary legible script, he lays the text flat on the table and looks into an upright mirror placed on the left or right side of the text. I shall always refer to the latter arrangement as "mirror writing," "mirror image." I shall refer to the other arrangement as "upside down." (See this also page 186.)

[9]They did not do this all haphazardly. The name ALEPH starts with an /a/ sound; both HÉ and KHET contain an E-related sound, and the /i/ sound is only half a vowel

even for us. Thus, YAD was a logical choice for /i/. How the AYYIN, meaning "eye" (the English and Hebrew words almost sound like cognates), became an /o/ I don't quite know. Certainly, our /o/ looks like an "eye."

[10]GAMMA is the third letter in the Greek alphabet.

[11]As for the /v/ sound which the Latins also needed, they finally had to satisfy themselves with the Greek UPSILON, which they adopted and used as both vowel and consonant. Its place is almost at the end of the alphabet. At present, the letter V serves as a consonant: /v/ in English, /f/ in Dutch or German. Of the two related letters U and W, one represents a vowel (= /oo/) and the other a consonant (= /w/), quite different from /v/ to the English ear.

[12]Those knowledgeable in Hebrew will be aware of the fact that the Hebrew letter PÉ has a different form depending on whether it falls within a word or at the end of a word. The form that suggested itself in this discussion is the word's-end version.

[13]I guess a child with brain damage simply finds it harder to learn, so that more time and greater effort are needed to teach him the shape and the directional character of letters. Writing has to be emphasized even more, and phonic rules ingrained with longer chains of paradigm words.

[14]Goldberg (1968) is one of the authors who clearly states that dyslexics might read "was" for "saw."

CHAPTER NINE

*On Consonant Crowding, Contour Crowding, and on the
"Hierarchic Order" in Communication by Language — A
Note on Alexia — A Note on Syllabic Writing*

I shall now turn to another common handicap I have encountered in
children with reading problems with great regularity, whatever the
cause: they become utterly confused when asked to read words with
"crowded consonants" *aloud.* And it need not be as many as three
or four consonants. For a poor reader, two consonants are often a
"crowd." To a certain extent at least this must be a physiological
difficulty, exaggerated in the poor reader but present in the normal
child. And it must have some phylogenetic background. Comparative
linguistics abounds in examples of vowel insertion or consonant ero-
sion, the purpose of which clearly must be the avoidance of some difficulty — otherwise the tendency would not show itself with such
regularity and in so many different language groups. Let me give as
an example a Slovak word taken over by Hungarian. Slovak is a Slavonic language. Hungarian is not. People who speak Slavonic languages apparently have no difficulty pronouncing crowded consonants. Their languages seem to thrive on consonants. The Poles call
a city known to us as DANZIG (four consonants to two vowels)
GDANSK (five consonants to one vowel). The Slovaks even have
words in which an L or an R (both of them so-called liquid consonants) supplants a vowel.[1] VLK means wolf in Slovak, KRK means
the throat, PRST, a finger. A word like KRČMA, meaning a country
pub, offers no difficulty to a Slovak. Hungarians got around to un-
crowding the consonants by inserting the vowel O between the consonants K and R.

156

In an earlier part of this book I gave some examples of the elimination of consonants in the French language. They happened to be examples of consonant elimination in the middle of words. Elimination of one of a crowd of consonants from the beginning of words, again particularly of the sound /s/, is almost the rule in the French language. Moreover, by adding the vowel E. the French managed to shift the originally crowded consonants away from the beginning of words altogether. Thus, the French created, to cite only a few examples, such words as

ÉTRANGER from EXTRANEUS (STRANGER)
ÉTUDE   from STUDIUM
ÉTAT   from STATUS
ÉTOILE   from STELLA
ÉCOLE   from SCHOLA
ÉCRIRE   from SCRIBERE
ÉPICE   from SPECIES (SPICE)
ÉPONGE   from SPONGIA

In these examples they both eliminated a consonant from and (except for the first example) added a vowel to the beginning of the word. In other examples, like

ESPÉRANCE from SPERARE
ESPRIT   from SPIRITUS
ESCALIER   from SCALA
ÉPROUVER from PROBARE

they did only the latter. An especially attractive example is

EMERAUDE from SMARAGDUS

where the French eliminated two real tongue twisters, SM and GD, from one word.

The Spanish are satisfied by the enveloping vowel without elimination of the consonant, as in

ESTADA   ESCUELA
ESMERALDA   ESTADIO

No such definite tendency seems to have emerged in English pronunciation. Only in words probably taken from the French or Spanish rather than the original Latin, as in

ESPOUSE   EMERALD

is an attempt to soften the initial syllable apparent.

As I said, this tendency to avoid consonant crowding (tongue twisters, we might call them) especially at the beginning of words must have some physiologic reasons. In the handicapped reader the inability to handle crowded consonants becomes almost pathologic, and often incapacitating. In the course of my routine diagnostic examination of children with reading or spelling difficulties, presentation of crowded consonants occupies an important place. So does oral reciting, which readily brings any difficulty in this area to the fore. I am most emphatically opposed to "silent" reading, or "sight" reading during the learning period. (These accomplishments come later, and they come automatically.)

Let me emphasize again: Letters are essentially symbols of sounds: written words are essentially symbols of spoken words.

As Geschwind (1972) has clearly stated, "the visual pattern [in reading] must first be converted to the auditory form before the [written or printed] word can be comprehended." This is the natural sequence of events. "Conversely," he continues, "the auditory pattern for a word must be transformed into the visual pattern before the word can be spelled." In neither case can the "auditory pattern" be eliminated. Its place is between "seeing" and "meaning."

Attempted short-cuts from "looking" to "meaning" (the aim of the "meaning" school of teaching) only magnify the poor reader's problem. And they merely hide or camouflage the difficulties children can have with crowded consonants. A child has to be able to pronounce these in words which are sequences of sounds before he can ever expect to master them in written sequence form. And he must be able to write them down in sequence before he can be expected to read them off the printed page. The process follows a strict order, almost a hierarchic order.

In my directives to parents (as I have indicated, I am a great believer in involving parents; I teach the parents how to teach their children), exercises with crowded consonants play a preeminent role, all based on my cluster technique. Exposure to problems of consonant crowding follows, in my method of teaching, right after the concept of the retroactive modifier has been introduced and understood, and often even before that other difficult phonic problem, digraphs, has been presented. In fact, the three routes of successful phonic practice generally intertwine, as is obvious from the clusters of examples of increasing complexity which I have given all through in this book. For the reader with good capabilities crowding of consonants represents no more than what seems to be some kind of a physiological difficulty, a difficulty easily overcome. However, in a minority of cases, in problem cases, the attack must be more systematic, using what I call the "lead word" or "prompter word" technique. As an example, take a rather easily mastered group of "lead words" all beginning, say, with R, and of appropriate "crowded" words all beginning with BR:

RAG/BRAG	RIDE/BRIDE
RAT/BRAT	RIGHT/BRIGHT
RIM/BRIM	RIDGE/BRIDGE
RED/BRED/BREAD(!)	ROOM/BROOM
RING/BRING	REED/BREED
RACE/BRACE	REACH/BREACH/BREECH(!)
RAKE/BRAKE	

I dictate such word pairs in random order and write them slowly on the blackboard. Hearing, copying (all this is done with written letters first; no printed text interferes!), loudly repeating them, the child familiarizes himself with the sound and sight of a "crowd" while at the same time he reviews previously learned material (the modifiers, the digraphs, the modified C, the modified G), revealing any weak points that need reinforcement by added examples.

In these examples there is only one challenge: a "crowd." Further examples, such as

RAW	BRAWN	BRAWL
ROW	BROW	BROWN

force the student to face more than one challenge at a time. (Note that in the last two words the sound of the vowel also changes.) Finally, he is given "unprompted" BR words (many of them familiar from other problem exercises):

BRED BREAD BRIEF BREAK BRINE
BRASH BRUSH BRICK BRACK BREAST BRAND

(the last two words with a "double crowd") to finish the lesson.

Another technique (to add variety and interest) is the presentation (by dictation!) of one or two prompter words with a string of crowded words (some of them unexpected):

LOW	INK	LACK
BLOW	LINK	BLACK
GLOW	BLINK	BLANK
SLOW	RINK	
	BRINK	

RIB	LOOM	RAKE
RIP	ROOM	BRAKE
LIP	BLOOM	BREAK
DRIB	BROOM	DRAKE
DRIP	GLOOM	DRAPE
GRIP	GROOM	DRAIN
GRID	GLOW	TRAIN
CRIB		DRUM
TRIP		DRUNK
TRAP		TRUNK
TRIM		
FLIP		

RIM	MILL	ROW
BRIM	MILE	CROW
GRIM	SMILE	GROW
FIRM	LIME	THRONG

ORE	RAID	HUT
TORE	GRADE	HURT
STORE	GRACE	HERD
SPORE	TRADE	SHERD
SCORE	TRAIN	HUSK
		DUSK
		DESK

An endless variety of pairs and strings can be set up by an energetic parent or teacher and adjusted to the individual pupil's potential, ranging from easy words, like many of those just given, to quite hard words, with three or more consonants crowded on one or both sides of a center vowel:

RAW	WRONG	REAM	LEFT
STRAW	STRONG	STREAM	CLEFT

RAGE	PRINT	SPRUCE
RANGE	SPRING	SPLASH
GRANGE	RING	SLIM
GRAND	SPRING	SLUR
STRANGE	STRING	SMITH
CRINGE	STING	SMART
SINGE	STRICT	STRENGTH
SING		

BEAR	VEER	SEAR	SEARCH
BEARD	WEIRD	SHEAR	BIRCH
			CHURCH

The possibilities seem endless, though in reality they are not. The teacher will do well to point this out. There are actually only a few consonants that crowd others — the R in:

BRUSH	CRAB	DRINK(!)	FRINGE(!)
GRIME	PROP	TRASH	WARM[2]

the L in:

BLOT	CLAM	FLOP	GLUM
KLING(!)	PLOT	SLOT	CALM

the N in:

BANG	BEND	TENT
LINK	RING	SONG

It is not just by accident that R crowds were our first choice in the first cluster of examples and continued to be the most common even among the examples that followed. R, a liquid consonant, *is* the most common crowder; L, another liquid consonant, is the next most common; N is not uncommon. They always stand next to the vowel, the R and L generally in the front half of the word (only occasionally at the end, as in WARM, CALM); N crowds are always at the end. Words like BRINK or KLING are crowded at both ends. M rarely crowds,

BLIMP   SHRIMP[3]

S is a case in itself: it is always the first in any crowd:

SPEAK	SPIN	SCRIPT(!)	SPRING(!)
SCUM	SLIM	SMITH	SNAKE(!)
SPEAK	SPIN	SCRIPT(!)	SPRING(!)
STRICT(!)	BEST(!)		

(SNAKE is no exception: the crowder is the S, the N is only one of the consonants crowded upon.) Words like

SCRIPT   TRACT   STRICT

are unassimilated, more-than-one-syllable Latin words. I am not sure we should consider CT or PT a consonant crowd. The fact that PNEUMONIA is pronounced without the P and KNIFE without a K shows that the English mouth and ears are also not fond of too many consonant crowds. (Note the pronunciation of such terms as PSY-CHOLOGY and PTOSIS in this connection.)

Once a child with reading difficulties has mastered crowded consonants, half the battle is won. But often this is a terrible task. (Some of the examples given are real tongue-twisters!)

I have digested a lot of literature on dyslexia over the years and it is amazing to me that the problem of crowded consonants is hardly ever broached. The degree of dexterity with which crowded consonants are handled is for me a principal, possibly the principal, diagnostic and prognosticating guide to the management of any patient with reading difficulties.

Psychologists will recognize a well-known phenomenon which is related in name only to the problem we have just touched upon. "Crowding of contours," as this phenomenon is often called, can, under certain circumstances (amblyopia is the foremost among them), interfere with recognition of letters in words. I will mention a simple experiment (Woodworth, 1938) to demonstrate the inhibiting or "masking" effect of one contour upon another adjacent in a line of print. If a person with normal visual acuity fixates from ordinary reading distance upon the center letter o in the upper row of Fig. 3a he is still able to recognize the letters t and s in spite of the physiologic amblyopia (poorer visual acuity) of the retinal periphery. However, as soon as these two letters are enveloped by other letters (as in the second row of Fig. 3a), the subject cannot recognize the letters t and

t   o   s

nte   o   hsx

a

o

bom

sbomk

asbomku

easbomkut

geasbomkutc

wgeasbomkutcz

dwgeasbomkutczh

idwgeasbomkutczhv

xidwgeasbomkutczhvp

fxidwgeasbomkutczhvpn

rfxidwgeasbomkutczhvpnj

yrfxidwgeasbomkutczhvpnjl

b

Fig. 3. Mutual interference or masking of letters in indirect vision. (a) Fixate the letter *o* in the upper row, and the letters *t* and *s*, on the left and right side, are clearly visible. Fixate the letter *o* in the second row, and the letters *t* and *s* become illegible though they occupy the same retinal position. They are *crowded out* by the surrounding letters. *(b)* Fixate the center letter *o* in this pyramid of nonsense words. You can bring your gaze down the line of letters *o* for a considerable distance and still recognize the first and the last letter of each line, even when the letters in-between have long ceased to be recognizable, and although they are much closer to the point of best vision.

s any more, although their respective distances from the center, and thus their respective positions on his (the observer's) retina, have not changed. Crowding, physical crowding of contours, has an inhibitory effect upon perception. Another simple experiment is even more convincing: We expose an observer's eye for a fraction of a second to increasingly longer nonsense words built of random letters, such as in Fig. 3*b*. (He has to fixate the center letter o.) We would expect that all the observer can remember having seen after such a short exposure are the three or four center letters upon which his gaze actually fell. The fact is that he also sees, and quite clearly remembers, the letters at either end of even rather long words. The explanation is obvious: these letters were the only ones not masked, not crowded out of perception, by adjacent contours.

This phenomenon is related to visual acuity. If, assuming he has normal vision, the observer turns his gaze to either of the three-letter groups (Fig. 3*a*, lower line) the masking effect (it is a kind of reciprocal inhibition) disappears. Only if the letters are very small, approaching the threshold of recognition in the fovea, will crowding of letters intefere with recognition of fixated letters. Improving visual acuity by proper correction (if feasible), by choice of print of appropriate size (if visual acuity cannot be improved), are therefore among the ophthalmologist's prime duties if he is faced with a reading problem. In this manner he can minimize the effects of contour crowding.

Reciprocal inhibition of letters in a printed text is, of course, to a certain extent, inevitable. Flom and associates have found (1963) that, if letters near the threshold of recognition are separated from each other by about 120 percent of their own width, there is no more masking effect, and that the masking effect is most pronounced when the separation is around 30 percent of the letter's width. Unfortunately, this is more or less what the separation between adjacent letters is in any ordinary type. No wonder, then, that the kind of reciprocal inhibition we are talking about might plague the beginner engaged in the process of learning to read. It is almost impossible to provide a child with printed matter that avoids this, and it would serve no purpose. Masking or no masking, books, magazines, and newspapers must crowd a maximum number of letters into the confines of the fovea, the area of sharpest vision, and a maximum amount of information into a minimum number of pages. Books would be too heavy and too expensive if the text were printed in a manner that avoids crowding. We ultimately learn to read quite rapidly and efficiently in spite of this. Only advertisers can afford to buy uncrowded attention space. Advertisers know that a newspaper page that is half empty carries its message more effectively than one filled with "copy." Compare the attention value of

A M E R I C A N

M E D I C A L

A S S O C I A T I O N

(separation more than 100 percent of letter width) with

AMERICAN
MEDICAL
ASSOCIATION

(separation less than one-third of letter width) to see the difference. And although in the example just given the individual letters are of identical size and occupy the same visual angle, the more separated letters can be recognized from a greater distance. Acuity of vision is not simply a matter of visual angle.

As I emphasized earlier (see Chapter Seven) our eyes stand still while our mind scans through a word or a cluster of words. Contour interaction is unavoidable under these conditions. The penultimate letters on either end, especially, are blotted into nonperception during the reading pause, the pause between eye movements during which all reading is done. When a poor reader struggles with

spring   strong

I sometimes have the feeling that he actually does not see some of the letters, especially the second one at either end. He reads *sring* or *sping, ston* or *srog,* frantically trying to find a word of meaningful sound. He wants to *hear* meaning, not see it! I cannot tell whether or not a poor reader would do better with uncrowded type in the early stages of study. It would certainly be worthwhile to find out.

As I mentioned earlier, I am an advocate of oral reading rather than silent reading in the early phases of the teaching-learning process, and I feel especially strongly about this in the case of the poor reader, whatever the cause of his difficulty. The poor reader (unless he is also mentally retarded)speaks better than he reads. And if he has been exposed to the "look-and-see" meaning technique, we can expect him to know many more spoken than printed words whose meaning he has successfully been taught to "see." His disability is strictly in the realm of "de-coding" printed words whose sound equivalents he may understand very well. He has not yet mastered the phonic approach. He has not yet built that two-way bridge between the "visual pattern" and the "auditory form."

I am also an advocate of teaching students to write before teaching them to read type is taken up in any systematic manner. As I pointed out in the previous chapter, it is through writing that we imbue letters and words with the directional qualities they must possess. In fact, reading comes about all by itself as the student follows his own hand or the teacher's hand while writing letters, writing words.

There is a strict, call it hierarchic, order built into communication by symbols. This order (the order in which we learn to use symbols to express thoughts) cannot be reversed and should not be tampered with. Speech comes first and reading last in the developmental history of systematized communication through symbols. At first, sounds had to become symbols of thoughts (to paraphrase Hobbes: *oratio* had to become the symbol of *ratio*) in the history of our race. Symbolic speech had to develop first. Only then could visible forms, patterns made timeless by some kind of writing (and I mean writing in the widest possible sense of the word), become symbols of these symbols.

This strict order (the "phylogenetic" order) repeats itself in the developmental history of the individual (the "ontogenetic" order). The time sequence uttering-listening (communication by the spoken word) precedes the time sequence writing-reading (communication by script) in the development of the individual as much as in the development of the race. Nobody can read before he speaks. Speaking stands between reading and thinking, and only via the spoken word will reading communicate thoughts.[4] We do not read thoughts, we do not read meaning, however rapidly and however silently we read. Let me repeat: the meanings belong to the sound! We only reinforce the meaningfulness of reading in the beginning reader or the retarded reader by interposing sound, actual speaking, between reading and meaning. Hence:

1. *Start with oral reading in every case!*
2. *Continue with oral reading in the case of the poor reader for a prolonged time!*

Time-sequence order, strict evolutional order is a principle we must constantly be aware of if we want to understand the neurophysiology (also the neuropathology) of a function as complex as communication by symbols, the language function.[5]

It was the great British neurologist John Hughlings Jackson (1884) who in his several papers on "Evolution and Dissolution of the Nervous System" first emphasized that neuropathology, and more specifically the mode of "dissolution" of neural functions, is a reliable guide to uncovering this evolutional order. Jackson's laws of hierarchic order (expressed in somewhat more up-to-date words) read about as follows:

> Phylogenetically (or ontogenetically) older function patterns hold out longest and recover first when affected by disease or injury; phylogenetically (or ontogenetically) more recent function patterns are lost or damaged first and recover last — their vulnerability is the greatest.[6]

And to this we might want to add:

> A disturbance that can occur in isolation earmarks a more recently acquired function pattern.

One can, to give an example, suffer from a defect or disarrangement of color vision, whether hereditary or acquired, without his light sense being affected. But one cannot have his light sense affected while his color vision remains normal. As a corollary to this, many species of animals, even of higher orders, possess only a light sense and no color vision. (It would be truly preposterous to assume the reverse.) Obviously, color vision is a "higher" or more recent "evolutional" acquisition: it can be lost in an isolated manner, while the appreciation of luminance, the light sense, is a more basic faculty, also a more ancient one.

Another example from the field of visual perception is stereopsis. One can well exist without it. It is a late acquisition. (A cross-eyed child will never develop stereopsis.) But there cannot be a person who has lost the retinal or other clues of space perception (the whole gamut of so-called monocular clues of depth-and-space perception) while achieving stereopsis.

To juxtapose spoken and written language in a similar manner is almost facetious. Certainly, spoken language is the older acquisition of the race, and millions of people still utter, hear, listen to, and comprehend "spoken" language without ever having known anything about its written form. There can be no question about the primacy of spoken over written language.

The hierarchic order, which manifests itself in symptoms lesions of the language function, merely confirms the primacy of speech. In fact, it was precisely through the application of Jackson's principles that Freud (1891) first brought order and system into the complex of syndromes going by the name "aphasia." I cannot enter into a discussion of this complex since only one facet of it, "alexia," is pertinent to our topic.

Alexia is "loss of *previously acquired* ability to interpret symbols or to read." According to Keeney (1969), alexia appears in three major neurological forms. The least grave of them is a condition called "pure alexia" or "alexia without agraphia" or "agnosic alexia." Appearing as an isolated lesion entity, this type of alexia is obviously indicative of the loss of a "young" function in the Jacksonian hierarchy.

Dejerine (1892) in one of his famous papers classified one of his cases as "pure word blindness with spontaneous writing and writing on dictation unaffected." This case obviously belonged in this group.[7]

The second of these three groups is comprised of a less restricted syndrome of lesions in the communication machinery; besides reading, it involves writing as well ("agraphic alexia"). Dejerine (1891) described one of his pertinent cases as "word blindness with agraphy or very marked disturbances of writing." A lesion in the so-called angular gyrus of the left side would cause such a syndrome. (Presence of such a lesion was verified by postmortem study.) Such a lesion would separate the visual association area from the auditory language area without disturbing the connection between the auditory area and the motor areas involved in speech. In other words, such a lesion would affect reading and writing but would leave intact the more ancient communication functions, speaking and listening.

It is only in the full-blown case of what is called Wernicke's sensory and motor aphasia that *all* language functions find themselves involved — the more ancient symbol categories as well as the more recent ones.[8] Both listening ("comprehension") and speaking as well as writing and reading are affected.

Knowing as little as I do about the history of the language function, I dare not discuss in earnest the question of whether listening or uttering came first in the early dawn of the birth of language. Possibly the question is not even justified — the two are much too interrelated. I suppose the same holds true of the two younger functions, writing and reading. Still, the fact that in "agnosic alexia" the ability to read is lost "without agraphia" permits one to state with some assurance that writing must be the older function. In any event, handwriting should be practiced before reading type is taught. And both should be actively reinforced as long as necessary by the even more deeply established modality of communication: uttering (and by its feedback control hearing one's own voice). Thus, oral reading should be cultivated.

These are the points I wanted to make.

I have just dealt with certain problems in the phylogenesis and ontogenesis of communication. Therefore it should not be unjustifiable to finish the chapter with some comments on the evolutional history of writing.

In a previous chapter, referring to the origin of certain Hebrew and Latin letters, I may have given the impression that a straight line of evolution leads from pictographs to the alphabet as a culture develops and that this evolution follows some simple principle of acrophony. For example, the letter A, the "picture" of an ox, came to be sounded /ah/ because ALEPH, the word for ox, starts with that sound; the letter B, the "picture" of a house, came to be sounded /b/ because BEIT, the word for house, starts with that sound; and so on. (A reversal of this principle is still in general use in our first-grade texts, which use the picture of, say, an APPLE to teach the sound and form of the letter A, the picture of a BABY to teach the sound and form of the letter B, etc.) But the impression would be a mistaken one. The Chinese, for example, never gave up pictorial writing, though there can be no question as to the depth and breadth of their civilization. There are other ways to develop a simplified script than evolving an alphabet. One of these is "syllabic" writing.

For the ancient Greeks (some of their tribes at least) syllabic writing was an interim step of development; they readily discarded it, in truly Greek fashion, when they met with the Semitic alphabet (one or the other of its several branches), which was much more adaptable and much better suited to their language and their purpose. But for the Japanese, syllabic script has remained a going means of communication up to the present day. We shall see why in a moment.

For the manner in which syllabic writing may have developed from the pictorial (ideographic), I can give no more attractive example than one I read in *Life* years ago.

This magazine (at one time — alas, no more) used to publish some extremely well written, popular, yet authoritative pieces on the history of our civilization. One of these was a piece dealing with the history of written language. (In order to understand the argument of

the imaginary story which I want to quote, we will have to make ourselves believe, for a moment, that the hero of that story spoke English.)

Let us then assume, according to *Life*'s imaginary story, that a
picture of a BEE, a sufficiently abstract symbol, in the course of time
became associated not only with the mental image of a bee but
(through innumerable recalls, simply through the length of the association) also with the spoken sound sequence *bee*. Let us also assume
that in the course of time a similar association developed not only
between the picture, the ideogram, of a LEAF and its mental image
but also, necessarily and through long association, between the ideogram and the spoken sound sequence *leef*. Now let us picture the
hero of our story, our reading-writing ancestor, struggling with the
task of putting into writing, in some manner, a concept he had developed and wanted to communicate, a concept the spoken word for
which happened to sound approximately like *bee-leef*. And now
imagine our ancestor suddenly realizing that he could put the ideogram for *bee* and the ideogram for *leef* next to each other in some order to be agreed upon to symbolize his concept. At that moment, the
two pictures are freed from the respective mental images which they
had represented up to that time. They now merely symbolize the
respective sound sequences *bee* and *leef* and, together, in an agreed
sequence (say from left to right), represent a concept, BELIEF,
which carries no mental image of any object associated with it.

At that moment the patterns put on paper or clay or whatever
changed from ideograms into phonograms, the written symbols of
sounds (as it happens in this example, the symbols of syllables),
symbols independent of the things which the pictures originally
represented. It was at that moment that writing with its present
connotations was born.

Yet whatever tremendous contribution toward an efficient writing system our imaginary hero made, his invention in the long run
would not turn out to be "economical." Let us for a moment imagine
a writing system in which the picture of a LEAF would be the symbol
of a sound sequence, *leef* or (to make it more basic and simple) *lif*.

Then let us realize how difficult it would be to find an appropriate and simple ideogram for all the possible variations of either of the
component consonants in this syllable,

lib	*lic*	*lid*	*etc.*
bif	*cif*	*dif*	*etc.*

Obviously, a system like this would be uneconomical in the extreme. The fact is that a language like Hebrew or English in which there are, word for word, generally more consonants than vowels cannot sustain economical writing on a syllabary basis. Think of examples like

MISH-MAR (in Hebrew)   STRENGTH (in English)

with four consonants to two vowels and six consonants to one vowel! However much I like *Life*'s story, what it describes would have been a wrong start toward the phonogramic writing of a great many languages. Syllabic writing could and did (except for "short" periods of experimentation, which in Mycenaean times could be centuries.[9]) stay only with languages in which, word for word, the number of consonants is either smaller than or, at most, equal to the number of vowels. Japanese is a good example of a great civilization that found syllabic writing a useful and efficient expedient[10] and we now understand the obvious reason: Japanese syllables either consist of just a vowel or of a single consonant plus a vowel (to which sometimes a "nasal" n, a kind of half-consonant, can be added). Thus, in

O-GU-CHI

there are three vowels to two consonants while in

HI-RO-SHI-MA   CHO-CHO-SA(N)

the number of vowels and consonants is equal (not counting the n in the last example). Assuming that in some language there are five vowels and twenty consonants (these are rather valid averages), one needs no great mathematical apparatus to find out that there can be no more than twenty-one "Japanese-type" syllables, e.g.,

a   ba   ca   da   fa   etc.

(in alphabetical order) in which /a/ figures as a vowel. The same will hold for the other four vowels.[11] In fact, if a paleographer finds that in some unknown script there are about one hundred different characters, then he can assume, with rather good certainty, that the script is syllabic and that the syllables are of the "Japanese" type.[12] On the other hand, a script in which there are about thirty characters must be alphabetic. An alphabet is the only viable ("economical") type of script for languages with consonants as the basis of word structure (Hebrew) or with consonants in overabundance (the Indo-European languages).

NOTES

[1]To a certain extent this is also true for English: In words like LIT-TLE, CAT-TLE, HUR-DLE the /l/ sound has a vowel-like value.

[2]In words like

FIRM   GIRL   MART   CHURCH

we can consider the R a crowder. But we can also look at it as a vowel modifier. One view reinforces the other.

[3]N and M can also be considered liquid consonants. It is their vowel-like character which makes it relatively easy to pronounce consonant crowds that contain an R, L, N, or M.

[4]Even the deaf-mute must be taught to intercalate "sound," a temporal sequence, between reading and meaning.

[5]I cannot help inserting a few paragraphs here which may be heavy going to readers unfamiliar with terms of neuroanatomy, especially those related to the language function. They can skip them without too much loss of continuity.

[6]The wording has been changed somewhat, since Jackson, in nineteenth-century fashion, spoke of a "hierarchy of nervous centres" even though he was obviously quite aware of the fact that what he actually was speaking about was *functions* rather than *centers*, if the word center means some kind of anatomical entity. The term "nervous centers" has by now lost much of its meaning. Geschwind, for instance (to quote one recent example), in an essay entitled "Language and the Brain" (*Scientific American*, April, 1972) speaks of *areas* (e.g., Broca's or Wernicke's area) rather than centers. He also rather refers to *anatomical locations* (e.g., the *angular gyrus* which "contains the 'rules' for arousing the auditory form of the [visual] patterns in Wernicke's area," or the *arcuate fasciculus* along which "the auditory form is transmitted [from Wernicke's] to Broca's area"). In Geschwind's remarkably lucid diagrams, connections from the visual cortex are strictly to the auditory. Nowhere is the existence of direct communications to higher brain locations (communications which dodge, so to speak, the auditory brain) even suggested. Neuroanatomy offers no indication for a direct route from "seeing" to "meaning."

By the way, Geschwind's paper, since it is in such an easily accessible publication, will be understandable even to those who know little of brain anatomy. No one interested in the reading problem should miss reading it.

[7]However, the detailed history of this case shows that the functional lesion was not truly isolated. The patient also had right-sided hemianopic amblyopia with loss of color vision in the same half-fields. Obviously, the anatomic lesion involved more than merely some hypothetical "reading center." Still, it left most of the communication machinery intact. Those interested will find an illustration in Geschwind's article that explains the underlying brain pathology simply and well.

[8]In Keeney's words, the following four disturbance categories are present: "incomprehension of spoken . . . language"; "incomprehensible and characteristic speech disturbance due to distorted or incorrect words and extensive circumlocutions"; "inability to write correctly"; "incomprehension of written language." In these patients, alexia is only one of the symptoms in a grave syndrome — Wernicke's aphasia.

[9]Those poor Mycenaeans, stuck with a syllable script for a while, would have written my last name as

li-ne-ke-se

in order to represent the sounds heard, even approximately. (No wonder they did not hold onto this type of script.)

[10]For historical reasons that may be interesting but are irrelevant here, the Japanese use Chinese ideograms as a basis and employ syllabic notations to solve some of the problems presented by this system of writing, which is essentially foreign to their language.

[11]According to a tabulation by Gelb (1963), one of the Japanese syllabaries contains five characters for the vowels a, e, i, o, u, respectively, 68 characters for simple consonant-plus-vowel syllables, and one symbol for the affixed nasal *n*.

[12]For those interested in the history of writing, the book *The Decipherment of Linear B* by Chadwick (1958), a paperback published by Random House, should be a genuine treat.

CHAPTER TEN

A Note on the Brain-Damaged Child — Is Bilingualism a Handicap? — A Short Autobiographical Aside — Reading Material Already Known by Heart — The Lefthander and Writing with the Left Hand — Lefthanded Musicians — The Right Hand Is the "Right" Hand — Problems and Difficulties of Writing with the Left Hand — Mirror Writing, "Upside-Down" Reading, Boustrophedon

I shall now return to some of the problems posed by the poor reader and shall start with a disclaimer. I am, I must confess, not qualified to make statements about the statistical share of brain damage in the complex generally presented under the heading dyslexia. I am also not qualified to diagnose minimal brain damage. I am sure that there are many children who suffer from the consequences of birth trauma, of maternal anoxia in some phase of gestation or parturition, or of premature delivery, or from genetic metabolic disturbance, etc. I am also sure that such children add to both the problems and the challenges of teaching reading. Not being connected with a large pediatric center, I have just not seen a sufficient number of cases in which I could satisfy myself that I was really in the presence of the syndrome so often and so loosely called "brain damage." Often I do see that young patients in my office behave in a manner in which children with so-called minimal brain damage are supposed to behave. Some children move around constantly, handle every piece of equipment, pay attention to each and every detail of the surroundings except the one they are expected to concentrate on and become extremely fatigued. I don't know how much of such behavior in poor readers truly stems from brain damage and how much represents secondary psychological superstructure.[1] The fact that really poor readers are mostly boys makes it unlikely that brain damage is a rather common cause of the disability. Brain damage should affect boys and girls with equal frequency. The same fact also makes it, I confess, difficult to blame all or most reading disabilities on poor teaching techniques. As I see it, satisfactory answers are not yet forthcoming, but the value of such a teaching technique as the one I have outlined in the foregoing chapters is independent of any theory on, or classification of, dyslexia. Teaching phonics is a must — it is not a matter of taste or choice — in the case of the severely handicapped reader.

I feel there would be no point in entering into the psychologic-psychiatric-sociologic complexities associated with dyslexia. A number of outstanding analysts have discussed its psychological aspects, and no less a man than James Conant (1964), at one time president of Harvard University, devoted a volume to the problems of *Slums and Suburbs*. I am the last person to belittle their work and their conclusions. Of course, my main concern is teaching. Slum children even more than suburbanites, brain-damaged children even more than geniuses, should be taught, I feel, to write and read (note the order of the words) by the phonics method. Let me repeat this: Teaching phonics is a must, not a matter of taste or choice, in the case of the handicapped reader.

But even if I don't think I could or should discuss any of the psychological aspects of the dyslexia complex or the significance of family upbringing and economic circumstances among its causes, I must, I feel, dwell on one related aspect of the problem, the question of bilingual upbringing, and voice a personal conviction. Perhaps the children of poor Puerto Ricans in city ghettoes or of poor Mexican-Americans in rural ghettoes are poorer readers, percentagewise, than the children of white Protestant or white Jewish suburbanites, but certainly not because of the former's bilingual upbringing. Bilinguality is, I am convinced, a blessing, not a handicap. A bilingual person (and here, aside from my own conviction, fortunately I can quote an authority like Professor Kolers of MIT[2]) has two sets of tools to solve a problem, not one. I am sure (I have tried to show this in foregoing chapters of this book) that this holds especially true for English spelling. The rules for English spelling cannot be understood, indeed must be utterly confusing, without some knowledge of other languages. I am sure that German, Latin, and Greek, which primary and secondary education forced upon pupils in the pre-World War I Austro-Hungarian Empire, helped, not hindered, my acquisition of English, that beloved and wonderful tool that I have now been using for almost half a lifetime.

Here in America, at least when my sons were small, bilinguality was considered a kind of handicap. It set a child aside from the idealized average. It was a blemish on wished-for conformity. It confused the IQ scores. Neither of my two boys passed the admissions tests for the Hunter College kindergarten school mainly because, at the time they were given the tests, they spoke better Hungarian than English (the language in my household is Hungarian), and this scored against them. The test was given to my older son at Columbia University Teachers' College, and I remember one item. When he was asked what a *bed* was, he did not give any explanation in English but said in Hungarian, "AZ EGY ÁGY." He obviously thought that giving the corresponding Hungarian word for the English word bed proved that the "concept" of a bed was not unfamiliar to him. He failed in matters of "conceptual thinking."[3]

Though in America bilingualism was, seemingly, frowned upon and is still given again and again as a cause of retardation in reading, for a Jew in the old Austria-Hungary it was natural to grow up in a veritable Babel.[4] In the town where I was born, I was constantly exposed to four languages. My father spoke German[5] at home and with most of his older co-religionists, he spoke Hungarian to the authorities, he spoke Slovak (a poor, not too literate Slovak) to the maidservant and the man who came to cut our firewood, and, finally, he spoke in Hebrew to the Lord. (He was a Rabbi and spent many hours of the day praying and studying the holy books.) And being a devout Jew, he followed the Talmudic instruction according to which a boy of three must learn to recite the daily prayers. I don't remember when and how I learned to write and read, it was so early in my life. I am sure it was my father who taught me and I know that by the time I got into first grade (I was just five years old) I was as fluent in speaking German as in Hungarian (Hebrew was studied and understood but never spoken). I read Hebrew, Hungarian (the Latin characters), and the old "black-letter" (we called it Gothic) script, the type that at that time was still in general use for writing and reading German. I still don't know if my father did right, but my father did know. He followed instructions whose soundness, sanctity, and validity he did not doubt. When many, many years later my younger son was given a so-called reading readiness test in the kindergarten class of Collegiate School in New York, the headmistress of the Lower School told me that the boy was "not ready" to read (he read Hungarian words into the letter combinations[6] he picked up in store windows along New York's East 86th Street) and I was forbidden *(expressis verbis)* to attempt to teach my child to read. He entered first grade a year later, unadulterated by any knowledge I could have imparted. The contrast was prodigious. Did *I* do the right thing?

In any event, from my earliest days, it was never unnatural for me to carry my gaze from right to left reading the Bible in Hebrew or from left to right reading the translation printed on the same page. The meaning of the type made this necessary. In other words, I learned to approach things from more than one angle, and I am convinced I have no strephosymbolia. I am also convinced that the signal contribution Central-European intellectuals have made to our new fatherland is at least partly due to their readiness to see things from more than one point of view. If we read reports like the one by Mme Fermi, the widow of the famed physicist, about the achievements of the so-called refugees, we need not be ashamed.

Spelling English intelligently requires some acquaintance with other languages. So there seems to me nothing unnatural in the fact that it was Flesch (1955),[7] an Austrian scholar, who made what I consider the most important breakthrough toward the sound teaching of English writing, reading, and spelling by exposing the fallacies of the "see-the-meaning" system.

I have never had the chance to find out if it really helps the poor reader to acquire some reading skill if one lets him read some text he already knows by heart. According to vaguely remembered conversations, this was the technique my father used in teaching me, probably without giving it much thought.

As a child I went with my father to the daily prayer services. I must have been very young when he started taking me. I don't remember when he started — just as I don't remember when I started or how I learned to write and read. (I suspect my psychoanalyst friends would have an explanation for this.) In any event, I must have known some daily prayers, some Sabbath songs, by heart at a very

early age. My father began every meal with a benediction. He chant-
ed a psalm (the One Hundred and Twenty-Sixth or the One Hundred
and Thirty-Seventh) after every meal and a whole string of them on
the Sabbath. I still know those psalms by heart, words and melody.
The cardinal statements of the Hebrew faith starting with

Hear, Israel: The Lord Our God Is One Lord . . .

I heard recited three times a day. It is this statement of faith that,
according to the precepts of his religion, a father must first teach a
three year old son. I am quite sure I already knew the words by heart
by the time my father first made me look at them in the prayer book.
Perhaps he just intoned a word at a time and then left me to my own
devices to match letter to sound.[8] (Leaving me to my own devices
remained his favorite teaching technique.) Perhaps, it would help if,
instead of the stories about Sally, poor readers were given to read, in
the version familiar to them,

Our Father who art in heaven
Give us this day our daily bread.

There might be a miraculous breakthrough, a revelation — the sud-
den realization of what seen symbols are actually standing for.
    Of course, the words could also be

London Bridge is falling down

or

The cow jumped over the moon

or, perchance,

O, say, can you see
By the dawn's early light

One could use anything known to the child as spoken text before he
has ever seen it in the printed or written form. This would be a kind
of inverted look-and-say technique, the matching of printed symbols
to sounds with meaning (in proper Jacksonian order) rather than the
other way around.[9]

    I have also tried another approach: I present the patient with a
cluster of words, say,

HAD, HAT, HID, HIP, HIT, HOT, HUT, HUNT, HATE
HASTE, HIDE, HOPE, HEAT, HOOD, etc.

and ask him which words he thinks matches the spoken word *hit* or
hāt or *hĭd* and give a rationale. I hope to create a connection in this
manner between a visual and an auditory image. (Unfortunately, I
have no occasion or opportuni y to try out such ideas on a group of
poor readers. I must leave them as suggestions for further studies.)

After this autobiographical aside, I want to return to the problems of poor readers and especially to clarify some points about
mirror writing and about writing with the left hand.

In our civilization, lefthanded people are at a definite disadvan-
tage. They read what, from their point of view, is essentially mirror
writing. What is mirror writing to us is natural writing to the lefthander. By the very nature of his motor endowment it would be easier
for him to write Latin letters (penned, not chiseled, Latin letters!)
from right to left. This is the way the lefthanded Leonardo da Vinci
wrote, unencumbered by teachers and, obviously, by the thought
that not many would bother or be able to read what he wrote. This
was his privilege.

But generally, people want their writing to be read. Thus, lefthanded or not, when taught the means of communication, a child in
our civilization must learn to write and read from left to right and *to
develop a system of ocular-manual kinetics*,[10] a system of vectors
which run from left to right, not only in the arrangement of words but
in the forming of every single detail of every single letter. A lefthanded child has to be taught to write (*and* read) the words

NEW YORK

in the manner indicated in Fig. 5b. Thus, while he is encouraged to
write with his left hand, he still has to write righthanded letters from
left to right. Under the guise of permissiveness we are actually using
sophisticated coercion. We teach a lefthanded child to write and read
in a way that to this child and for the left hand is not natural. We are
not doing the lefthanded child a favor by letting him write with the
left hand. Lefthanded people, had they been in the majority, would
have developed individual letters designed for the left hand. They

would write from right to left writing English and (strange as it may seem) from left to right writing Hebrew or Arabic. In other words, they would have developed a kinetics of vectors and an arrangement of symbols that are the mirror images of the one we righthanders have developed. As things stand now, lefthanded children, even when permitted to use the left hand, must learn and are taught to write righthanded English letters (from left to right, the way we righthanders do it) while teachers, educators, and psychologists nurture the illusion that these children are left "free" to develop "unwarped left-handed personality."

No one so far seems to have noticed (or made note of) the fact that lefthanders cross their t's from right to left while writing from left to right. To me, this indicates conclusively that they write under constraint and will assert their lefthanded personality wherever they find a loophole, a chance.

As far as the training of lefthanded children is concerned, I feel that every reasonable effort is justified in trying to redirect them to write with the right hand. As I mentioned earlier, I have never yet seen a violinist hold the bow in the left hand, although I am sure there are lefthanders among violinists. (I am told Charlie Chaplin does, but this would certainly be an exception that confirms the rule.) If holding the bow in the right hand can be forced upon the lefthanded, I don't see why holding a pen or pencil cannot be.[11]

I have recently learned that Professor Rudolf Kolisch of the New England Conservatory of Music bows the violin with his left hand. However, according to information furnished by a Boston newspaper, Professor Kolisch was not born lefthanded. He suffered some severe injury to the left hand (the one supposed to do the "fingering") as a child, and it would have been necessary for him to give up a promising musician's career had he not switched the bow (and, I assume, also the strings). Obviously, here is a man who, under the compulsion of circumstances, and under the guidance of wise parents carried the role of the "aggressor" over to his nondominant hand (and his nondominant brain hemisphere?).[12] There is no reason why it should not be feasible to carry the skill of writing over to a nondominant right hand, since, as far as language function is concerned, the chances are that the child is left-brained anyway.

Recently I saw a painting by the nineteenth century American artist William Sidney Mount (1807-1868) at the Whitney Museum in New York (Fig. 4). It is the portrait of a violinist. The young man holds the instrument and fingers it with the right hand, the bow is in

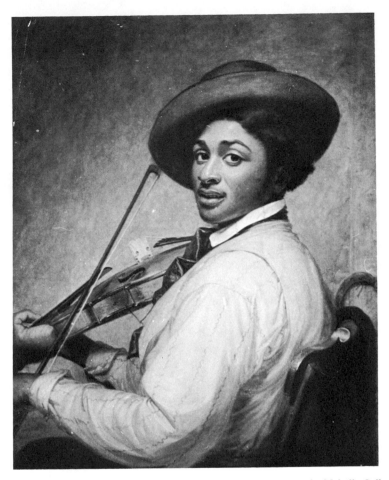

Fig. 4. Right and left. A painting by William Sidney Mount in the Melville Collection of the Suffolk Museum. (Reprinted with special permission of the Suffolk Museum at Stony Brook, Long Island.)

his left. It is the only realistic painting of a lefthanded violinist I ever saw.

The title Mount gave the picture was *Right and Left.* The title is authentic. Mount kept a careful *Catalogue of Portraits and Pictures* which has been preserved. Obviously he was conscious of the problem presented. (Mount himself was an accomplished musician, and there are several portraits or pictures of players with their instru-

ments among his *oeuvre*.) Mount's catalogue mentions that the painting was made "for the House of Goupil & Company to be engraved
in Paris." The exhibition catalogue adds: "When the picture was
lithographed in Paris, it was copied directly onto the stone; conse-
quently, in the print he plays like a proper violinist." Thus, it seems
that Mount's painting is not really the portrait of a lefthanded
violinist.

In the Metropolitan Museum in New York, among a series of
Manet masterpieces, there is a portrait of a young Spanish-looking
guitarist shown plucking the strings with the left hand. He must have
been a genuine lefthander.

A fifteenth century tapestry altar frontal now in the Cloisters in
New York depicts *The Life of the Virgin* in several panels. In one of
them, "The Coronation of the Virgin," one sees an angel plucking a
guitar-shaped instrument with the left hand. However, it was obviously not meant to depict lefthandedness, since many other details
show confusion of right and left in the panel: God, the Father, gives
his blessing with the left hand, and Christ, who is supposed to be
seated *ad dextram Dei Patris*, occupies the left side.[13] In another
panel, "The Visitation," Mary and St. Elizabeth shake left hands on
meeting, etc. Obviously, the tapestry weavers did not worry about
whether the finished work was the mirror image of the cartoon after
which it was patterned. They did not mind depicting a lefthanded
angel or God giving his blessing with the left hand.[14]

To play the guitar with the left hand (and have the strings re-
arranged accordingly) is, it seems, not a great rarity. But, I have never
seen or even heard of a "mirror image" piano for a lefthanded pianist.
I have never learned of a lefthander reading music from an inverted
sheet, nor have I ever heard of a lefthander who would write the
mirror image of

$$\flat\kern-0.5em\text{♪} \qquad \text{or} \qquad \flat$$

The fact that after a leftsided brain injury suffered at an early
age, a child can learn to speak again, suggests that originally both
brain halves have some language capabilities and that, if the occasion
arises, the right brain may prevail. The experiments of Professor
Penfield, the famed Canadian brain surgeon, conducted during
operations on conscious patients, corroborate the assumption that

the appropriate areas of the right brain have or retain some voice forming (though not speaking) capabilities even in the adult right-hander. On the other hand, when it comes to expressive language, then, according to statistics of Goodglass and Quadfasel (1954), even lefthanders are left-brained: lefthanders too become aphasic following injury to the left brain in the overwhelming majority of cases. And, of course, even lefthanders have their heart on the left side.

Visual images from the left field of vision fall upon the right visual brain cortex. (See Appendix A for reasons and details.) But (according to Geschwind's analysis of Dejerine's case of "pure" alexia) when it comes to "seen" language (written or printed matter) then, via a special radiation of nerve fibers, these visual impressions arriving in the right brain must be channeled to a "visual language interpretation area" (the angular gyrus) on the left side. We were not told by Dejerine that his patient was righthanded but we can, with some confidence, assume he was. And in view of the statistics by Goodglass and Quadfasel, we can with similar confidence assume that the visual language interpretation area even of lefthanders will be preferably localized in the left brain.

In conclusion, we are not doing any prima facie harm or damage if we try to redirect a seemingly lefthanded child's writing. We are doing a child an injustice if we let him develop into a lefthander if he shows only slight indications of a left choice. We don't have to be so permissive. We don't have to be so guilt-ridden. Our civilization is a civilization of the right hand, the aggressor hand, and we cannot change that.

By the way, much of what is called brain damage, confused laterality[15] faulty egocentric localization, belated development of hemispheric dominance, etc., in the lefthanded child is sheer, induced schizophrenia. *We* create the problem, not the twisted brain symbols. *We* let the child write with a hand that he constantly hears is "not right." "Right" means "correct" in American usage. For a German the word *Recht* means the "law." For a Spaniard *derecho*, for a Frenchman *droit*, is "straight" and "righteous." The word *pravo* in Slavonic languages is related to *pravda*, the "truth." In Hungarian, significantly, *jobb* means the "better" hand.[16] (The English homophones I discussed earlier only add to the schizophrenia. The lefthanded child is permitted to *"rīt"* with a hand that is not "*rīt.*") We exclude the child from the brotherhood of the "correct," the "lawful," the "upright," the "true," the "better." We let him belong to the "*gauche*," the "*sinister*" instead of the "*dexterous*," and, adding insult to injury, we don't even let him write in a way natural to him. Why are we so afraid that we twist a child's personality? Are we not doing just that?

From my own experience I must confirm the generally held opinion that there is a greater percentage of poor readers among lefthanders than among righthanders. Is the poor ability to read really caused by the same twist in hemispheric dominance that caused the lefthandedness? Or is it not just a secondary outcome of the way we handle or mishandle the lefthander? I am almost afraid to ask a lefthanded six-, seven-, or eight-year-old youngster: "Which is your right hand?" What should he answer? He would love to hold up his left hand; after all, that is his *correct* hand, his more *dexterous* hand, his *better* hand! He hesitates. He gets confused. And just look at his poor parents! Their agony shows in their tightened face muscles. They think I think their child is a moron because he had to think, and because he hesitated. And that my verdict will destroy any hope of their child's ever learning to read, because it is now proved that the child's brain is damaged. Then I give the child a pencil (it is almost always a boy) and ask him to write his name. Many of these poor lefthanders have not yet learned how to hold a pencil in the left hand, how to rotate the page to enable them to write those righthanded letters with the hand that isn't "right." It is all artificial schizophrenia, induced by teachers who teach nothing but "Look-Sally-Look," by parents who want their lefthanded child to "develop his own personality," by all of us who let lefthandedness prevail when probably it could easily have been changed.

Of course, I may be biased. Coming from Central Europe and belonging to the generation of elders, I have many lefthanded patients and friends who were forced to write with the right hand in school. I don't know if in any way they became more unhappy, more handicapped, more twisted in their ambitions, more frustrated in their personal relations than true righthanders or lefthanders left to their own devices. Does anyone know?

If we let lefthanded children use the left hand for writing, at least we must be aware of the difficulties. The main problem is the formation of the individual letters since they evolved through the use of the right hand. This hardship has fortunately lessened since round hand with pen and ink went out of vogue, and especially since the introduction of the ballpoint pen, a writing tool without inherent directional features. The difficulty is reduced still more if the child is permitted to rotate the page so that the writing flows from upper left to lower right, the natural direction of strokes for the left hand. A young ophthalmologist who is lefthanded told me not long ago about the agonies he suffered in school when learning to write with the left hand, since his teacher insisted that the pad of writing paper be held straight on the desk. Obviously, this teacher had no understanding of the special problems that face the lefthanded child during the process of learning to write *our* way. She only knew the rules, and all she cared for were her own ideas about tidiness and discipline. I feel it would be better to use proper coercion all along. If the right hand is the "right" hand, the "better" hand, the "dexterous" hand, why not use it for writing? If coercion is necessary, why not all the way? But if a child *is* permitted to write with the left hand, then he needs special instruction, special guidance, and a teacher who knows the problems this child is facing The teacher must be aware of the fact that the letters the child is going to write are righthanded letters. She must know that only through the proper holding of pen, hand, and paper will a lefthander ever achieve a reasonable flow of ink, of lines, of letters. Lefthanded people naturally draw their lines from upper left to lower right. Thus, lefthanded children have to be taught (or left along to teach themselves) to write from upper left to lower right, not straight across, and especially not from lower left to upper right.

Recently I had a severely confused lefthanded boy in the office. He was nearly eight years old and almost a total nonreader. When I asked him to write his name, he took a pencil in his left hand and held it in his fist the way one usually holds a dagger. He could not possibly see the point of the pencil as he made an attempt and was utterly lost in the mechanics of his procedure. His parents were completely unaware of his difficulty. Obviously, they never thought of analyzing how their son held a writing utensil, and the teacher seemingly never bothered to watch or instruct him. She either didn't know or didn't care.

Before I conclude this line of thought, let me once more refer to that most familiar visual pattern, the two words:

NEW YORK

Figure 5 shows these seven letters (printed capital letters) in an

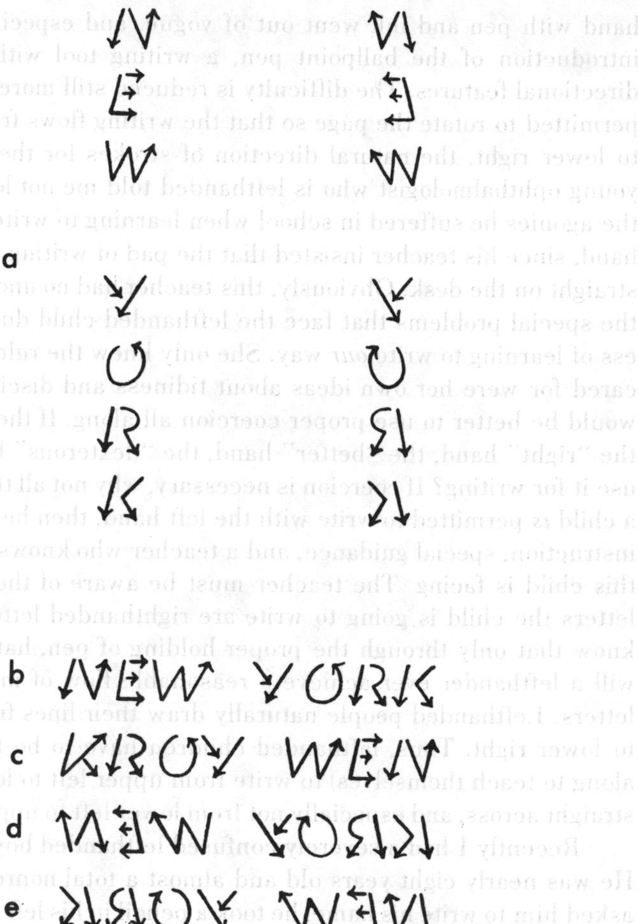

On Writing, Reading, and Dyslexia

Fig. 5. Right-left problems in the arrangement of strokes within letters and of let-ters within words. (a) The characters follow the Chinese style, running from north to south. The letters in the left column are righthanded letters: the individual strokes run and also follow each other from left to right. The letters in the right column are "mirror" letters. *(b)* The righthanded, "normal" Latin arrangement, i.e., left-to-right oriented letters follow each other from left to right. For righthanders, the majority, this is the best possible arrangement. *(c)* The letters have retained their righthanded, left-to-right character but follow the "Hebrew" arrangement in words. *(d)* The imaginary case of the "lefthanded Hebrew" is shown: lefthanded letters run from left to right. *(e)* Ordinary mirror writing, the best possible arrangement for a lefthander writing Latin letters (especially Latin script).

order running from north to south to eliminate, for a moment, the purely conditioned compulsion of reading along some particular horizontal direction. The letters in Fig. 5a are given twice: on the left, they are printed as they would be by the right hand; on the right, they are printed as they would be by the left hand (in the mirror image). To emphasize the kinetic nature even of printed letters, each letter is made up of a series of arrows — a feature that is self-explanatory.

Actually there are four different ways to make a horizontal word sequence from these two sets of letters, as each set could, theoretically, start from right or from left.

Our usual choice (writing from left to right with the right hand) turned out to be the best choice; and writing two-component letters with the left component first (see, e.g., the letters N, R or K) also is a better choice, since this avoids smudging of clay or ink. This gives us the familiar pattern shown in Fig. 5b.

Let us now imagine a group of people who, for whatever reason, though writing righthanded Latin letters in righthanded style with the right hand, choose to do so from right to left. This would result in the somewhat absurd-looking word picture shown in Fig. 5c. This word picture is meaningless to me because through conditioning, I cannot help reading normal-looking Latin letters from left to right. (The paradigm child who read W-A-S for S-A-W certainly showed more imagination or flexibility than I can muster. He gave meaning to a word he could not master in the customary way by reading it backward.)

We will now imagine the following: A people with a lefthanded majority has developed a system of letters suited for the left hand while still, for some reason, deciding to start from the *(for them)* less advantageous side, i.e., from left to right.[17] These sorts of lefthanded Arabs or Hebrews would produce the word picture shown in Fig. 5d. *My* gaze inadvertently wanders over this sequence of lefthanded Latin letters from right to left, since I cannot help feeling that that is their natural order, but no meaning emerges.

Of course the most logical way for this people with a lefthanded majority would be to write lefthanded characters and to start writing on the right, as shown in Fig. 5e, so as not to smudge their clay tablets. Their easily executed and entirely logical writing would produce a mirror image of what is a natural pattern to us. As I have mentioned, Leonardo da Vinci wrote in this manner.

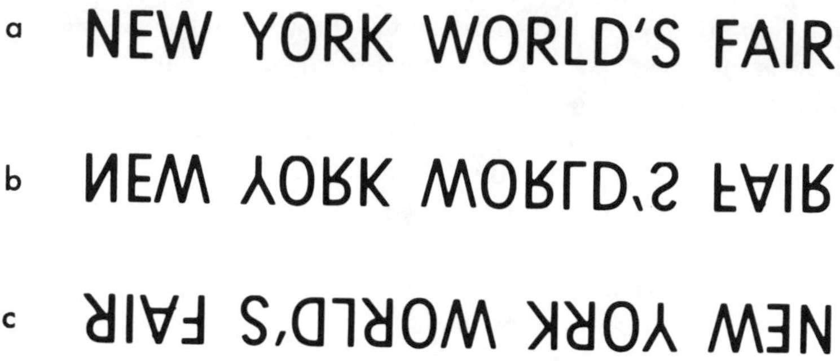

a   NEW YORK WORLD'S FAIR

b   ИEW YOЯK MOЯ⅃D,Ƨ ЬⱯIЯ

c   ИƎM YOЯK MOЯ⅃D,Ƨ FⱯIЯ

Fig. 6. *"Upside-down" image and "inverted" image. (a)* Normal Latin print. *(b)* "Upside-down" image of line *a.* There is no change in the left-to-right orientation of words, of letters, or even of details within letters. (See, for instance, the letters R or S.) *(c)* "Inverted" image. Note that the image of line *a* on our retina looks like the image in line *c.* It is "inverted," not "upside-down." Only if a mirror is held parallel to the row of letters in line *a* (above the line!) can one get an "upside-down" image such as shown in line *b.* Furthermore, note that this "upside-down" image is a "virtual" image. In contradistinction, the inverted image is "real": it can be projected on a screen. If line *a* is projected through a lens on a screen, the result is line *c*, and not line *b.*

On rare occasions (I know of only two cases) a lefthanded child may prefer to turn the printed page 180 degrees and read from right to left, in the direction best suited to the lefthander. This phenomenon has caused some confusion in the literature and has been described as "upside-down" reading, which it is not. The terminology is unclear. A mirror held parallel to (and above) a line of normal letters will give an "upside-down" mirror image, with the text still read from left to right, as seen in Fig. 6*b.* (This is the correct use of the term "upside down.") What the two lefthanded youngsters I have mentioned saw was something quite different and is indicated in Fig. 6*c.* The letters in this case are not "upside down"; they are "inverted," as is the retinal image. "Inversion" permits the arrangement of letters within words to remain congruous with the original, whereas a line of words and its "upside-down" mirror image are incongruous, as are all mirror images if one compares them to the original. Reading "inverted" print is not too difficult, even though one reads from right to left. Reading "upside-down" print is very difficult, although the direction of the reading continues to be from left to right. It is to be hoped that authors in the future will keep the essential difference between "inverted" and "upside down" clearly

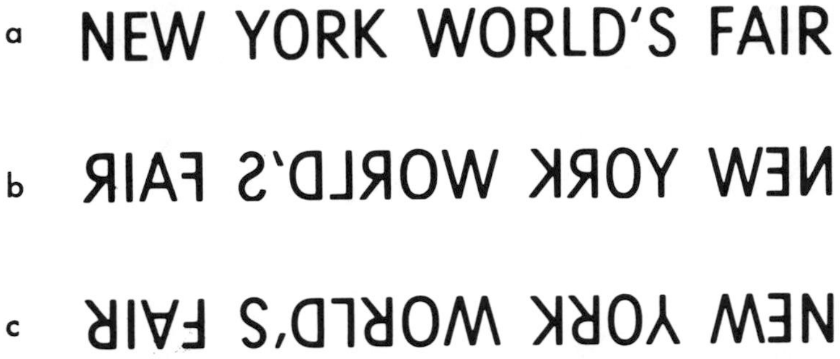

a NEW YORK WORLD'S FAIR

b ЯIAꟻ Ꙅ'ᗡⱢЯOW ꓘЯOY WƎN

c NEW YORK WORLD'S FAIR

Fig. 7. "Mirror" image and "inverted" image. (a) The words consist of right-handed letters arranged from left to right (normal Latin print). *(b)* "Mirror" image of line *a.* If the majority of people were lefthanded, presumably Latin print would look the way this line does: the letters would be upright, leftward oriented, and follow each other from right to left. *(c)* "Inverted" image of line *a.* If line *a* is turned 180 degrees one gets line *c,* and *vice versa.* Turning will not reinvert line *b* to regular print: only a mirror will do it.

in mind and will report accordingly. Rather than let confusion prevail, I shall once more present what I think we should call the "mirror image" and the "inverted image" of a printed line (Fig. 7). In both Figs. 7*b* and 7*c* the reading goes from right to left, as is best suited to a lefthander's manual kinetics and kinetic memory.[18] Figure 7*b* is the way Leonardo would have written a line in printed capital letters. (The way he actually wrote script is suggested in Fig. 9*b* and shown in Fig. 13, p. 202.) It is the way every lefthander would write if he had the choice, he himself being a mirror image of the righthander in terms of right and left, while both righthander and lefthander carry their heads *on* their shoulders. Note that the lefthander is not an "inverted" copy of the righthander. They are each other's mirror images in terms of a perpendicular mirror facing either of them.

In an extremely rare condition called *situs inversus* (I have only read about it in medical textbooks), the heart is on the right side, and the appendix, I guess, on the left. Obviously, the term *inversus* is used erroneously.

Figure 7*c* shows the "inverted" image of the printed line. Its advantage for a true lefthander who avails himself of it for reading is

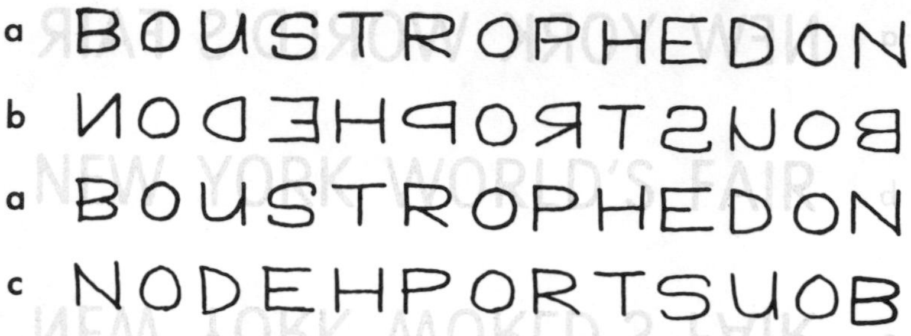

a BOUSTROPHEDON
b ᴎODƎHꟼOЯTꙄUOꓭ
a BOUSTROPHEDON
c NODEHPORTSUOB

Fig. 8. Boustrophedon ("turning like oxen" plowing): writing alternate lines in opposite directions. The two alternate lines *a* run from left to right; the lines *b* and *c* run from right to left. Line *b* is a regular "mirror" image of *a*: not only are the individual letters within the word arranged from right to left, the letters themselves are "mirror" letters, as if this had been done by a lefthander. In line *c* the individual letters retain their righthanded ("normal") directional structure; only their arrangement (from right to left) follows the path of the "turning oxen." This is essentially the Hebrew arrangement: individual letters are the righthander's letters but the arrangement of letters in words is from right to left. Lines *a* and *c* also remind us of the way in which the Japanese arrange written material. The Japanese have retained the original intrinsically directionalized, righthanded architecture of their individual written characters (whether they represent words or syllables). But the order in which they arrange these characters is open to choice (at least in modern Japanese). They can follow each other either left to right or right to left.

(1) that reading starts on the right and (2) that it is available. One just has to turn any ordinary print 180 degrees.

Turn this figure around 180 degrees. Line 7*c* will appear normal. You have reinverted an inverted image. In contradistinction, line *b*, the mirror image, will appear as an upside-down image. Mirror images and upside-down images are, in terms of geometry, incongruous with the real order of things (also they are "virtual" in terms of optical theory), whereas any object, including print, and its inverted real retinal image are congruous patterns. I am sure no lefthander in his "right" mind will ever try to read upside-down print in a parallel mirror from left to right.

I might raise a question here about *boustrophedon*, the ancient form of writing in which one line ran from left to right, the next from right to left, etc., in an alternating manner (Figs. 8 and 9). Assuming that the writing was done with the right hand the question arises, "Did the individual letters retain their right-handed identity, as suggested in line 8*c*, even though the text ran from right to left? Or by any chance did both the lines and also the individual letters turn the Leonardo way, as indicated in line 8*b*?

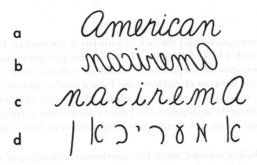

a *American*

b *American* (mirror writing)

c *nacirema*

d ‏| כ ֹ ר ֹ ל א כ |‏

Fig. 9. Attempts at boustrophedon with cursive Latin letters. The letters join easily
if the writing is from left to right, as in line *a*. They join each other just as easily in
mirror writing in line *b*. However, as line *c* demonstrates, it is impossible to write righthanded cursive Latin letters without interruption, without lifting the pen, if the direction of the writing is from right to left (boustrophedon) and if the individual characters
retain their righthanded inner architecture. Line *c* reminds one of Hebrew cursive.
Individual Latin cursive letters are righthanded letters: here they follow each other
from right to left, and therefore the pen must be lifted after each letter, often even
within letters. Line *d* shows the word "American" transliterated into cursive Hebrew.
(The word starts on the right.) The essential identity of the Latin and Hebrew characters is obvious even to one who does not read Hebrew.

A diagram in Diringer's book (1962) presents only the latter alternative. It certainly
is not the only possibility. The Japanese don't write *boustrophedon*. They don't alternate the direction of lines. But I am informed that they have the freedom to arrange
their characters in either direction, right to left or left to right. (They are great emu-
lators and, under Western influence, more and more they tend to arrange their characters, at least in medical and scientific publications, in horizontal rows from left to
right. This makes good practical sense, since algebraic formulas, graphs, and charts
are usually printed with Latin letters and Arabic numerals.) Still, the individual picto-
grams and syllabograms retain their original intrinsic structural character, whichever
way they follow each other. The arrangement reminds one of the situation suggested
in Fig. 5*c*, which shows Latin letters written in the wrong order, from right to left, but
letters which *individually* retain their original directionalized character. In any event,
there are two alternatives in *boustrophedon*.

   In the actual history of writing *boustrophedon* must have represented only a short
intermezzo. All it could have saved was the time it takes to carry one's gaze or one's
writing utensils from the end of one line to the beginning of the next. (If boustrophedon
were used in inscribing the deeds of an ancient king on a mountainside with hammer
and chisel there would, of course, have been quite some saving of time or effort.) There
would certainly have been no advantage as soon as script became cursive. Figure 9
gives an idea of the problems cursive script would have to face to utilize *boustrophedon*. Figure 9*b* shows the type of cursive script the lefthander Leonardo used. For a
lefthander, it is an excellent arrangement. The arrangement shown in Fig. 9*c* certainly
has nothing to recommend its use, even to a lefthander.

NOTES

[1] I have often suspected that the lack of authority in the modern American family has much to do with a lack of discipline. I suspect that just the opposite, the almost overwhelming presence of unquestioned authority (father's word = God's word) mirrors itself in the behavior of children (and I see a good number of them) from the orthodox Jewish, especially the Chassidic, ghetto. Many of the children in this inbred population are extremely nearsighted. But I don't ever remember having seen one with a reading problem. To me, the shyness, the inhibitedness of these children is almost frightening.

[2] Professor Kolers reported about his experiments with bilingual students in the March 1968 issue of *Scientific American.*

[3] Jews, gypsies, Armenians, Syrians, and Levantine Greeks are generally bilingual or multilingual, for centuries-old reasons — historical, sociological — which I cannot discuss here. All these people cultivate a kind of "intra-clan" language (and cultural heritage) besides the "environmental" tongue (and civilization). The Ladino of Sephardic Jews, the Yiddish of Eastern European Jews are typical clan languages. That there is a great and beautiful literature in the latter tongue does not alter this fact. It is a mistake to hang the epithet "lingua franca of the Jews" on either of them. A lingua franca, like pidgin English, serves (makes possible, makes easier) communication between different civilizations. Yiddish is strictly for communication within the group — a *Shtetl* language, a ghetto language written with characters unknown to the outsider, even written in the wrong direction. (I will be forgiven by members of the just mentioned groups of people if I remind the reader that pickpockets, impostors, fences, and professional thieves also have a kind of language of their own and that many of them are multilingual.)

[4] I was pleased when twenty-odd years later the very same institution gave my son first a master's degree, and then a doctor's degree in education.

[5] "Westernized" Austro-Hungarian Jews preferred High German to Yiddish, the jargon (as we called it condescendingly) of the Eastern Jew.

[6] He spoke the word in Hungarian when he saw the letters C-A-R-S in a salesroom window. The letter combination was a sort of ideogram to him.

[7] The well-known author of *Why Johnny Can't Read.*

[8] Note the important stipulation, "matching letter to sound." It was not "matching word to meaning." Sound and meaning were already known to me.

[9] I realize that there is very little a child nowadays is expected to learn by heart. It is not the fashion. It does not fit into the reading-for-meaning concept and our hectic drive through life. I think this is a pity. In the case of the handicapped reader, it is more than that. It is a serious omission. Like the blind, the handicapped reader must develop the capacity for retention through auditory channels. In terms of the Adlerian education principle he has to make a virtue of a fault. He can achieve amazing feats of retentive memory by training, and he should learn by heart that which is worthwhile learning by heart, which can only help him toward such a goal. I know two prominent surgeons who, in spite of severe reading disabilities, went through medical school with honors. They employed colleagues as readers. They always stayed *au courant* with their profession by going to meetings and listening to lectures.

I have lately made some tentative experiments in "pre-reading" some short stories to a fourth-grade reader. The remark, "I don't know this word" or "I have not yet had that word," definitely occurred less often when I asked him to "re-read." There was a kind of familiarity and a happy matching, on occasion, of printed with remembered words where otherwise there would have been a blank wall of noncognition.

[10]To my pride and sorrow, I discovered that this idea too has been described by Freud (1891).

[11]Actually (and this is an added hardship on the lefthander), the essential details of letters are vectorialized not only from left to right but from lower left to upper right. The letter elements or complete letters we were taught to write in school all ran in that direction, the natural direction for righthanded writing. Lefthanders cope with the problems in several different ways.

[12]Professor Kolisch permits me to mention (personal communication) that he writes with the right hand, cuts his meat with the right hand, and in World War I handled a rifle like any other soldier. He played tennis with the left hand. (This I find natural. He also holds the bow with his left hand. It is his "holder" hand.) In many things he is ambidextrous. He has some difficulty in deciding which hand or which side is meant when people refer to the "right" or "left" hand or the "right" or "left" side. While driving a car, he gets confused when told to make a "left" turn. He has to think, even look at his own hands first: the one he feels he would hold the bow with is the "left."

[13]In a painting which depicts the same scene (it dates from around 1400 A.D. and is in the Boston Museum of Fine Arts), one angel plays the violin and another the guitar, and both are righthanders. Also, God the Father gives his blessing with the right hand, although Christ sits on his left side.

[14]In a book in preparation entitled *An Ophthalmologist Looks at Art and Artists*, a chapter I have included deals with tapestries and graphic artwork in which the depicted subjects act "lefthanded" because the executors have inadvertently copied a righthanded cartoon or sketch. I also plan to discuss Raphael's cartoons for tapestries and Breughel's drawings for the engraver. Obviously, these great artists wanted to have the final product "right," just as Mount did. Thus, they made their subjects lefthanded in the originals they prepared for copying.

The problem offered by self-portraits is just what one would anticipate. The artist must look in a mirror to see his own features, and if he paints what he sees he must portray himself as a lefthander. More often than not, painters of bygone centuries used all kinds of tricks to avoid this appearance. Good examples are the Rembrandt self-portraits in Dresden, Paris, and San Francisco, or Velásquez' self-portrait in his famous *Las Meninas* in the Prado. In all of these, what appears to be the right hand but actually is the mirror image of the left hand carries some kind of painting or drawing utensil to give the impression of right-handedness.

[15]See the footnote on Professor Kolisch.

[16]Strange as it may sound, the Greeks used the word *aristeros* for "left," a word obviously stemming from *aristos* for "best." The Greeks had strong beliefs in the magic nature of names, in placating evil by calling it good. They called the Black Sea *Euxinos* (meaning "hospitable") just because they found navigating it so dangerous.

[17]When a lefthander uses hammer and chisel to sculpt rather than clay and stylus

to write (with the hammer in the left hand), working from left to right would actually be the more natural way to do it. (A lefthanded God would have written on his stone tablets in that fashion — lefthanded letters running from left to right — assuming, of course, that he wrote in Hebrew.

[18]See the case history of two lefthanded artists in the next chapter.

CHAPTER ELEVEN

Left and Right in Western Art — Chinese Script — The Lefthanded Artist — Lefthanded Warriors — Natural Selection and the Left Hand

In this concluding chapter I want to make a few remarks on art, Western and Oriental, and Chinese script, and add some observations regarding the artist's use of the right or left hand. I trust that none of these topics will be found irrelevant to the subject under discussion. As far as the first two are concerned, again I claim the privilege of the amateur. I have never made a serious study of either, and all I say may already be known to experts. For me they were exciting discoveries.

In a lecture given before the American Hungarian Medical Association (Linksz, 1965), I showed reproductions of two paintings on the same subject, a procession of blind men, one by Pieter Breughel, the Elder, and the other by Hokusai, the great Japanese. I used the Breughel to illustrate the observation that action (the procession of the blind in the example) is, in Western works of art, generally directed from left to right, with the story's consummation at the extreme right.[1] In the second example, the work of an Oriental artist, the opposite seemed to be true: the scene moves from right to left. I have since found an even more convincing example of this in the Medico-Historical Museum in Budapest, an illustration in an old Japanese medical text of the gradual growth of the fetus in its mother's womb from conception to delivery. The event is illustrated in a series of ten monthly steps, starting with conception on the *right* side of the panel. A Western medical illustrator would have devel-

195

oped the sequence starting from the *left*. "Serial" representations (e.g., the tapestry with scenes from *The Life of the Virgin,* mentioned in the previous chapter) have been favorite and ubiquitous subjects as church decorations for centuries. The "story in scenes," it seems to me, almost always starts on the left (it does in the example of this altar frontal) and proceeds toward the right.[2]

In the *Annunciation,* one of the favored subjects of religious art, Gabriel, the messenger, the "action carrier" in the painting, is usually depicted standing or kneeling on the left and directing himself toward the right, while Mary occupies the right half, the more important half, of the picture space. I could cite dozens of examples in the National Gallery, the Metropolitan Museum, the Cloisters. Strangely, we find the opposite arrangement in several of El Greco's *Annunciation* panels. But El Greco, for all his Italian apprenticeship, was not a Westerner. The El Greco arrangement also prevails in engravings and tapestries of earlier centuries for purely technical reasons: engravings and tapestries are mirror images of the artist's original. Accordingly, in the "Annunciation" scene of the tapestry "serial" *The Life of the Virgin of the Cloisters* mentioned earlier, the Angel Gabriel occupies the right half of the panel, and he also gives his salutation with his left hand.

The reason for the left-to-right arrangements in Western art is sufficiently obvious. It is a matter of conditioning. Pictures are to be "read." *We* start reading on the left. The *Orientals* don't seem to have this type of eye training. I don't know whether they generally start individual stories on the right. I also don't know if their serial paintings start, as a rule, on the right and progress toward the left. (Interestingly, some Chinese gallery owners whom I asked in San Francisco did not know either. They had never given it any thought.) The few examples I have had a chance to see certainly did go from right to left.

Even in totally nonobjective paintings, such as some of the masterly works of Jackson Pollock, I can quite definitely recognize whether the artist proceeded from left to right, using his right hand to throw the paint. (In his mature years Pollock seldom used a brush.) The curves, contours, lines, sprinklings, run from left to right. (One cannot actually "hang" a Pollock upside down, though some detractors of nonobjective art like to say this. One would destroy the kinetics of the work.)

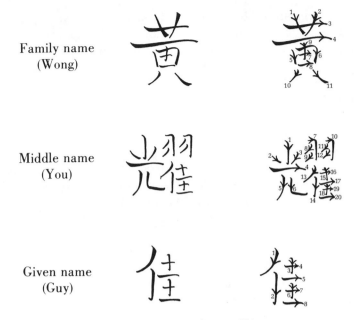

Family name (Wong)	
Middle name (You)	
Given name (Guy)	

Fig. 10. The three ideograms that make up a Chinese proper name.

Let us now turn to Chinese script. Recently I had the pleasure of holding a seminar with the fellows of the Smith-Kettlewell Institute of Visual Sciences of the Pacific Medical Center in San Francisco, and there I met a young Chinese-American ophthalmologist who, I am glad to say, has lost neither the language nor the script of his heritage. When I asked Dr. Wong to write down and analyze his name in Chinese characters he produced three ideograms (Fig. 10), the ideogram at the top being his family name, the one in the center his middle name, and the one on the bottom his given name. He worked with the right hand, holding the pencil as we would hold a brush. I asked him to repeat his procedure several times and carefully watched and followed every single stroke. He wrote the three ideograms from the top downward and nearer the right edge of the paper. (Had there been more text to write, the columns would have followed from right to left. Chinese individual characters — they are ideograms, not phonograms — are meant to follow each other from top downward, and the columns of characters run from right to left.) However, every single stroke was patently a right-hand stroke and, significantly, the horizontal strokes were always drawn from *left* to *right*, tapering off toward the right. Moreover, the individual strokes *within* each character also followed each other from left to right (also, of course, from top to bottom), and in both the middle and the given name, which have a kind of columnar structure, the left column was executed first! Clearly then, Chinese writing, as demonstrated by these examples, is righthanded writing, and it truly starts on the left in order "not to smudge" (my young friend used the term "smudge" unsolicited by me) the ink while it is still wet. ("The ink dries up by the time a column of characters is executed from top to bottom, and the next column can be started further to the left.") He also told me that the Chinese caligrapher will not rest his hand on the paper while executing his strokes with the brush. To me all this was an amazing and gratifying discovery.

In order to help me demonstrate more clearly what I mean, Dr. Wong redrew his name characters with some additions. Arrow markers indicate in what direction the individual strokes were drawn, and the numbers indicate the order in which they followed each other (Fig. 10). Obviously, these ideograms are kinetic patterns executed in a strict temporal as well as spatial order. The reader "sees" in them the kinetics of his own hand, the memory of his own muscular effort. Dr. Wong told me that he would be unable to jot down the strokes in any other order. He would be unable, he told me, to start his middle name with stroke number 20 (the last stroke) and then work his way backwards; or at any rate he would only be able to do it with great mental effort, imagining, so to speak, the finished product and working on what he saw with his mind's eye. Dr. Wong assured me that all the other characters he knows are written in a similar manner, and that he can produce them only if he holds to a strict order of individual strokes through which the picture "evolves." He could never produce any character by putting down individual strokes in random, reversed, or even different order. He also agreed that horizontal strokes are always drawn from left to right and that the *intracharacter columns* follow the same order. He was good enough to redraw and label for me some of the elementary characters of his language which I happened to have memorized (Fig. 11).

My knowledge of some of these characters stems from reading a popular essay, *The Triumph of the Alphabet*, by Moorhouse (1953). I don't remember that this author ever mentioned the fact that a Chin-

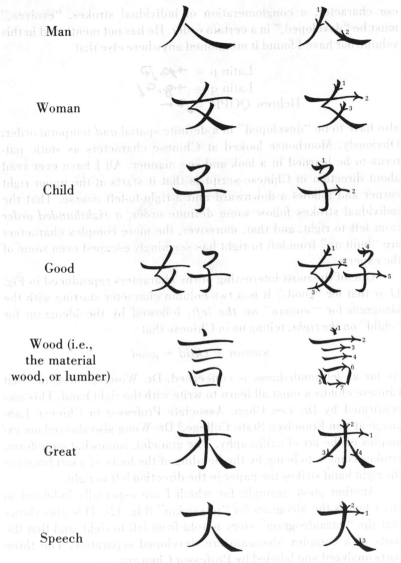

Man

Woman

Child

Good

Wood (i.e., the material wood, or lumber)

Great

Speech

Fig. 11. Some interesting Chinese ideograms.

ese character, a conglomeration of individual strokes, "evolves," must be "developed," in a certain order. He has not mentioned in this volume nor have I found it mentioned anywhere else that

$$\text{Latin p} = \quad \text{Latin q} = \quad \text{Hebrew QOPH} =$$

also have to be "developed" in a definite spatial *and* temporal order. Obviously, Moorhouse looked at Chinese characters as static patterns to be learned in a look-and-see manner. All I have ever read about direction in Chinese script is that it starts at the upper right corner and follows a downward and a right-to-left course. That the individual strokes follow some definite order, *a righthanded order* from left to right, and that, moreover, the more complex characters are "built up" from left to right has seemingly escaped even some of the experts.

One of the most interesting of the characters reproduced in Fig. 11 is that for "good." It is a two-column character starting with the ideogram for "woman" *on the left,* followed by the ideogram for "child" *on the right,* telling us in Chinese that

woman + child = good

As far as lefthandedness is concerned, Dr. Wong assured me that Chinese children must all learn to write with the right hand. This was confirmed by Dr. Leo Chen, Associate Professor in Chinese Language at San Francisco State College.[3] Dr. Wong also showed me examples of the art of calligraphy. The graceful, somewhat cuneiform, strokes come into being by the bending of the hairs of a soft brush as the right hand strikes the paper in the direction left to right.

Another good example for which I am especially indebted to Dr. Chen is the ideogram for "physician" (Fig. 12). This also shows that the "intraideogram" story is told from left to right, and that the parts of a complex ideogram are developed separately. The three parts analyzed and labeled by Professor Chen are:
1. Wound with arrow in it (top left).
2. Extracts foreign body with instrument (top right).
3. Treats wound with tincture (bottom).

Be all this as it may, Chinese script is, if anything, an argument against the look-and-say technique. I must conclude that not even

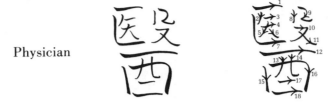

Physician

Fig. 12. The Chinese character for "physician."

Chinese ideograms are static look-and-see pictures, seen instantaneously and without a directionalized scan over their details. Chinese "ideograms" have to be produced and perceived kinetically and, as it turns out, from left to right, just as our and the Hebrews' righthanded letters are.[4] As I now see it, *Chinese characters are "melodies,"* true *Gestalten*[5] ordered in time as well as in space. They are not just "patterns." The individual strokes have to follow in an order that is temporal as much as it is spatial. Chinese characters have to be learned "by hand," certainly not "by eye" alone.

Finally, let us look at the problem of the lefthanded artist. As I have mentioned, lefthanded people naturally draw their lines from upper left to lower right. Leonardo, that most famous among left-handers, wrote his notes in mirror writing with the left hand, and as an expert on handwriting can tell he also drew with the left hand. This is evident from drawings in which he applied parallel or cross-hatched lines to give the effect of shading or relief. These lines run conspicuously from upper left to lower right. A good example is given in Fig. 13, in which one also sees his letters following each other from right to left. One might, of course, think that this is incidental or required by the design. The constant and unchanging character of Leonardo's cross-hatching lines is, therefore, more convincingly shown by his sketches of horses, a subject that intrigued him very much. In some of his drawings, a horse stands facing us, in others they are drawn facing toward the right or left. But in all of these examples, the cross-hatched lines run from upper left to lower right, independent of the rest of the outline. For contrast one might want to study a drawing by Rembrandt. Here, the shading lines run from upper right to lower left. Obviously, Rembrandt was a righthander,[6] (See Fig. 14.)

Watercolors are almost as instructive as drawings if one wants to study an artist in action since the aquarellist must work fast. One can

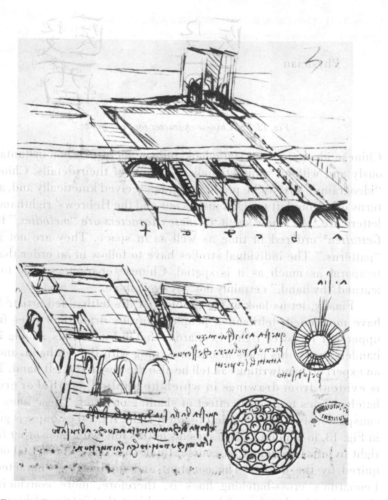

Fig. 13. Two drawings by Leonardo da Vinci. These drawings from Leonardo's *Notebooks* ("City Plans") show his way of mirror writing, and also the direction(\\\\\) of the cross-hatching he used to indicate shadows. It is interesting to note that the basic pattern of both drawings consists of quadrangles slanting to the left. Subconciously Leonardo used lines sweeping from upper left to lower right to outline his main designs: such lines were obviously easier for him to draw. The left half of the lower figure, by the way, is quite inaccurately drawn. The slanting lines are parallel and therefore appear to diverge: they do not run toward a common vanishing point. (Courtesy of The Bettmann Archive.)

tell whether the artist used his right or left hand by the way he laid dripping colors on paper with a soft brush. In Cézanne's exquisite watercolors (one cannot, alas, show these well in reproductions) both the pencil marks of the outline and the dabbings with the brush run from lower left to upper right. One can actually see how the pigment sagged under the influence of gravity while still wet. It is no wonder that an art lover loves drawings and quickly colored sketches. Studying them, he can almost feel he is in the presence of the artist, can see the artist's hand at work. (Formal paintings hardly ever convey such intimacy.)

An intriguing example, and at first glance an exception, is another work by Rembrandt reproduced in Fig. 15. We see the conspicuous cross-hatched lines once more running from upper left to lower right. Did Rembrandt by any chance use his left hand? He certainly did not. What this figure presents is the reproduction of an etching, not of a drawing. As is well known, for technical reasons etchings are mirror images of the artist's handwork. Rembrandt was righthanded. He drew his cross-hatched lines from upper right to lower left. What we see is the mirror image.

Rarely have I gained as much insight into the working of hand and mind of the lefthander as by watching a young, quite successful friend and patient, a commercial artist, at the drawing board. His designs for posters naturally contained some "copy" which he sketched into the design in the usual manner, from left to right, and of course with the left hand. As he explained to me, it is only by writing or reading text from left to right (as we all do) that the spelling and the words make any sense to him. However, once the design in, say, pencil, has been executed,[7] and what he called the "surface artwork" with brush and paint began, my friend started on the right side of the board and proceeded toward the left. "I abstract myself completely from "meaning" he said, and concentrate on form." Only in this way (for him the only natural way to fill in the outlines of a design) could he be sure of uncluttered brushstrokes with no likelihood of smudging. And only in this manner could he continuously survey what he had already done. What was most amazing to me was the fact that, as far as my friend could remember, none of his teachers in the High School for Industrial Design, where he had studied, ever remarked

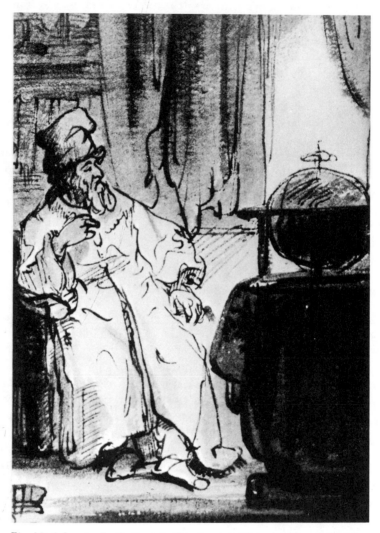

Fig. 14. A drawing by Rembrandt. This drawing *(Philosopher in His Study, Meditating Globe)*, shows the direction *(//////)* of cross-hatching characteristic of a right-hander. (Courtesy of The Bettmann Archive.)

on this duality of performance. It must be a rather common occurrence.

Another lefthanded commercial artist solved the problem somewhat differently. He, too, sketched the text material in from left to right, since that, naturally, was the way he had been taught to write and read. But for the artwork on the text, he turned the sketch "upside down." Having thus actually *inverted* the pattern he then proceeded with the brush from right to left which on an inverted text meant that he could work on the letters in their proper sequence. He did not have to abstract himself from meaning.

There is another question which, I think, still needs some airing. It is a justified question: if the dominant use of the right hand is biologically determined and subject to the laws of natural selection, why are there still some 8 percent of people lefthanded? Orton (1937), in his classic treatise *Reading, Writing and Speech Problems,* posed a similar question. He too was puzzled by "the persistent appearance of left-handed individuals of all races" and saw the explanation in a "hereditary tendency" asserting itself "in spite of . . . strong social pressure toward the right hand."

In attempting to answer let me turn to a subject I am more familiar with and look at the phenomenon of color blindness, an aberration from the normal whose preservation is negligibly affected by influences of environment, of upbringing, of "social pressure." Let me, then, ask the question: If normal color vision is biologically determined and subject to the laws of natural selection, why are there still some 8 percent of men (the percentage also happens to be 8 percent) who are color defective?[8] To answer it I should like to use a parable.[9]

Imagine a country, a grassland in some Arcadia, where Man and lion, eternal adversaries, have both survived since time immemorial. The grass is green, the lions are red, and if a man is color normal (able to tell red from green), then his chances of survival are considerable. With his skill and spear he will even be ahead of the game. Obviously, those who cannot tell red and green apart will have much less chance to kill, even to survive. If Darwin's so-called struggle for existence alone were operative, should one not expect that in the course of millenia Man would become color normal and all the lions extinct?

However, the Lord is not the keeper of Man alone. In his infinite wisdom he also created lions. And having created lions, he has some responsibility for their survival, too. This, the Lord's responsibility, is what we call the ecologic order of Nature, the order that maintains all species in remarkable balance, whether Man or beast. It is this Goethean striving of Nature toward balance that keeps most men color normal, some of

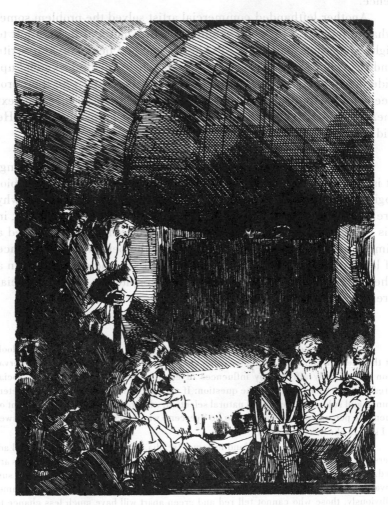

Fig. 15. An etching by Rembrandt. In this (*The Entombment*, first state) the cross-hatched lines run from upper left to lower right, being the mirror image of a right-handed artist's actual drawing on the copper plate. (This kind of conspicuous cross-hatching can best be studied in early sketches; in later states of this etching, the direction of the individual lines is hardly discernible.)

them (an amazingly constant percentage of them), color defective, and (in spite of Darwin) both Man and lion, as species, preserved.

This parable, however frivolous, has some modicum of truth, and one may expect a similar answer to the question, "Why are some people lefthanded in a world in which righthandedness has a biologic advantage and must by now be established as a hereditary trend?"

Again, my answer is somewhat facetious. If two primitive tribes were fighting each other for overlordship in some territory, and if all their men were righthanded, wars would never come to an end. A break in the deadlock could be expected only if there existed a certain percentage of lefthanded warriors who, while exposed to greater danger, at the same time had the advantage of thrusting their spears at an unusual and unexpected angle.

Variety and variability serve, as Dr. Kalmus has suggested, the ecology of Nature. The maintenance of a small percentage of aberrations from the normal may sometimes have some biologic purpose, and defeat in battle is not always the gravest of calamities. A reasonable peace treaty might ensue.

I do not know much about baseball, but I am told that a good lefthanded pitcher is worth his weight in gold, and that a lefthanded batter must then be found by the competing team to offset the advantage presented by the southpaw's unusual pitching.

The formidable, even ferocious, character of the lefthanded warrior must have been a known fact to the ancient. There are two references to it in Judges, probably the oldest and historically most authentic book of the Old Testament. The first one is to one Ehud, the son of Gera, a Benjamite, "a man left-handed" whose exploits on behalf of his fellow countrymen are given in such gruesome detail (Judg. 3:15 ff.) that they could not have been invented. The other reference is, strangely, again to members of the tribe of Benjamin. It is worth quoting (Judg. 20:15, 16):

> And the children of Benjamin were numbered at that time out of the cities twenty and six thousand men that drew sword . . . Among these people there were seven hundred chosen men left-handed; every one could sling stones at an hair's breadth, and not miss.

In combat that was not hand-to-hand, these men (significantly, some 3 percent of the warrior population) must have had the same advantage as our lefthanded pitcher.

As long as I am on the subject of the Old Testament and lefthandedness, I want to quote one more passage that, I confess, caused me some concern (Eccles. 10:2):

> A wise man's heart is at his right hand;
> But a fool's heart at his left.

Was wise King Solomon such a poor observer of anatomy? Or are wise men really that rare? In any event, this is the first suggestion I found in the "literature" linking the right hand to the heart. (Originally, I wanted to use this quotation as a motto for this chapter. Then I desisted. After all, most of us have our hearts "at his left." And we don't like to be called fools.)

　　　Lefthandedness may have some advantage some time, somewhere, and it is going to stay with us like color blindness. It is not just a "habit" that can be broken. It is a trait and, I believe, one with a hereditary background. One can, as the example of my two artist friends proves, accommodate his life and work to it. One can, as the example of Professor Kolisch proves, even train oneself to it. But it need not be cultivated. As I said earlier, we are not doing our left-handed children any favor by letting them write with the left hand. Unless weighty evidence to the contrary is presented, I shall keep on suggesting to parents that reasonable fortitude (not force) be displayed in shepherding a child toward the use (at least for writing!) of the right hand.

NOTES

[1] It was originally made by the famous Swiss art historian H. Wölfflin (1952).

[2] I found the opposite to be true for some church murals depicting *The Stations of the Cross*. There must be some reason for this which only a church art expert will know. Comic strips are, by the way, modern adaptations of the serial paintings. Their "story in scenes" also runs from left to right.

[3] I should like to express my thanks to Professor Chen for his kind cooperation and interest.

[4] Note once more that in the Hebrew cursive word depicted in Fig. 2 the horizontal embellishments of the letter g and the letter l both run from left to right.

[5] The German word *Gestalt* (plural *Gestalten*) is a noun meaning "something formed, a form." (Nouns are capitalized in German.) The word *gestalten* can also be a verb meaning "to form." *Gestalten* are "formed forms," not "patterns." Being "formed forms," Chinese characters carry the memory of their formation no less than our letters do.

[6] Books on drawings by great artists are easily available. It would be impossible to reproduce more of their work in this volume.

[7] He sketched a design to accompany the words

NEW YORK WORLD'S FAIR

[8]The 8 percent applies only to white males. In some more primitive races the number is smaller. There are, for instance, almost no color-defective males found in the Fiji Islands. Natural selection in the case of the Fiji has seemingly almost totally eradicated the color-blind.

[9]The answer was suggested by the reading of delightful books by the eminent geneticist. H. Kalmos (1964,1965), on color vision and some general problems of heredity.

APPENDIX A

Why Are We Righthanded and Leftbrained? — Why Do the Optic Nerves Cross? — Why Do the Motor Nerves Do the Same?

Two statements made quite early in the course of my discussion (both in Chapter One) necessitate, I feel, some further clarification. Both were rather loosely connected with my main topic. Therefore, neither could be elaborated at that time. I said: "We write with the right hand because our heart is on the left side," and after having heard me say this some of my friends thought I meant it to be no more than a witty remark for an after-dinner speech. I also said: "When the right hand became the hand of skills, the left brain had to become the matrix behind these skills." Let us now take a closer look at these two statements, and at the second, which is more important, first. In retrospect, was I justified in making it at all? Can we say that we are leftbrained because for some reason we are righthanded, as I in fact believe and as my sentence implies? May we not be righthanded because we are leftbrained?[1] Which is the cause? Which is the effect?

The real question, of course, is (if we are in the mood for asking questions pertaining to fundamentals): *Why is the left brain the*

· · · · · · · · · · · ·

This appendix is essentially a part of the introductory lectures on visual physiology which I have given for the past twenty years to future ophthalmology residents at New York University. Some of my lectors and advisers have found this appendix "too technical," as originally written. In the present version I have therefore tried to eliminate technical terms, and have added some rather elaborate footnotes and a kind of a built-in glossary.

210

matrix (the master) behind the right hand's skills? Wouldn't things
have been simpler had the Creator made the left brain govern the left
hand? There must be a reason behind what is seemingly such an
uneconomical arrangement. It cannot be just some poorer choice
perpetuated. Why, in fact, must the motor nerve tracts cross?[2] Why,
to make things even more complex, do the motor tracts to the lower
extremities originate from more coronal aspects of the motor brain
area and those for the upper extremities from more caudal parts?[3] A
clear answer to this was first given by Cajal (1898): *The pyramidal
tracts cross because the retinal images are inverted.* I can lean on
Cajal's authority in making this statement; it is not the expression of
an ophthalmologist's megalomania. I almost hear some of my readers
saying: "Imagine that tiny one-ounce receptable and the majesty of
the brain!" However, this would be an entirely unjustified interjec-
tion. The significance of the eyes cannot be determined by avoirdu-
pois. The retinas contain several hundred million sensory cells, cells
to catch the impact of light. But what is more important: each optic
nerve brings about one million nerve fibers (neural message carriers,
carriers of the information furnished by light) into the brain, and this
is more, counting nerve fibers, than those in all the other eleven so-
called cranial nerves together![4] Imagine that each optic nerve fiber
has its own "local sign": stimulation of it determines the location of a
point in seen space. Imagine one million light bulbs going on and off,
independently, on an advertising display board. What a wealth of
information about the space that surrounds the eye is available at the
spur of a moment! (The simile is, of course, exaggerated, since retinal
elements work in teams, as conglomerate sensory units, not quite the
way independent, individual light bulbs would on a display board.
But that does not really matter.) Imagine one million nerve fibers
from each eye carrying message elements from the surrounding
world into the brain. In any event, the question relating to the crossing of the motor pathways is a much more fundamental one than that
relating to the dominance of right hand or left brain. Dominance of
one hand, of one brain hemisphere, is a problem restricted to the
human species with its aggressions, skills, articulations, and problems of communication, while the crossing of the motor tracts is (so
far as my knowledge of these matters extends) a universal law of
neuroanatomic structuring throughout the zoologic division called
vertebrates.

Why should or how can the inversion of the retinal image have anything to do with this? To answer this question, I must take the reader along a guided tour. I must say a few words about the geometry of image formation in the eye, about the relation between objects in visible space[5] and their images on the retina, the inside lining of the eye, and about the possible ways of the transference (via nerve fiber tracts) of the retinal images to the receiving brain. Only then can I turn to the question of the relationship between the brain retina, as I shall call it, and the motor structures whose job it is to grasp, repel, or modify the objects of the visible surround under the guidance of vision.

The eye, at least the vertebrate eye, is a camera, a box with a hole (the pupil) and a light-sensitive layer (the retina) lining its back. Cameras "take" pictures, and so does the eye. Objects in the visible surround "form," as we say, images on the retina, and these images and the objects maintain a strict geometric relationship to each other. The relationship is best made visual with the help of a system of so-called polar coordinates.[6] The vectors of this system, of the eye's natural coordinate system, are the so-called visual rays,[7] lines that connect the objects with their images on the retina. All these visual rays pass through the eye's pupil; all of them cross each other in the pupil (more accurately, in the center of the pupil). Thus, the pupil is the natural pole of our system. One of the rays that enter the eye perpendicular to the plane of the pupil (specifically, through the center of the pupil) is the natural axis of the optical system of the eye, the so-called principal visual ray. It is the vector in the eye's polar coordinate system to which we can with the least compunction assign the distinctive value of zero inclination. It is the natural polar axis of our system. The object O in Fig. 16 from which this ray originates projects its image upon the natural center of the retina, the fovea. Every other point (that is, object in visible space) sends its visual ray toward the eye's pupil at some angle, at some definite and measurable angle of inclination which is different from zero. Each ray maintains this inclination until it reaches the retina. Thus, the location (or at least the direction) of any particular object in visible space and the location of its retinal image are characterized by a common inclination value usually expressed in degrees. By the way, the principal visual ray also has a biological as well as a geometric distinction. The principal ray, in addition to coming from an object straight in front

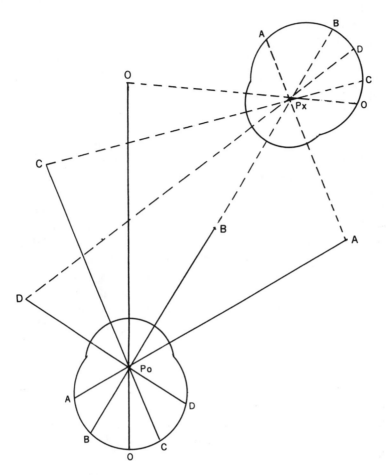

Fig. 16. The geometry of seeing: the simple geometric relation between objects in visible space and their retinal images. An array of points *A, B, O, C, D,* in "visible" space stimulates the retinal points *A, B, O, C, D.* The retinal locations of these points are determined by the position and orientation of the eye and by the so-called visual rays, or lines which cross in the eye's pupil, say at P_0. If the eye is oriented in the way shown in the lower half of the diagram, the ray from *O* will fall upon the geometric center *O* of the retina. The point will appear straight in front and will also be best seen, since the fovea, the area of best vision, is located in that region. If the eye changes its location in the space of these objects (if the pupil moves to P_x), and if it orients itself as shown, then the distribution of the retinal images becomes different: another point, *B* in our example, might appear straight in front and might also be best seen.

of the eye and rather accurately situated on its geometric axis, falls
upon a distinct and distinguished point on the retina, we have just
called it the fovea ("pit"), the built-in supersensor of the eye, the
area of best-detailed vision. Our tendency to relate all other object
points in our visual space to this best-seen object point of zero inclination is again a natural, an almost predictable feature of space perception or (to use a more general term) of spatial localization.
We call the direction of the best-seen object the principal visual
direction. The direction of any other object is given to us by the inclination between its visual ray *and* the visual ray to which we have
assigned zero inclination. The perception of the "relative" direction
of seen objects (right of center, left of center, etc.) is, in other words,
purely a matter of retinal geometry. No other clues are needed.

Now assume that an eye is exposed to object points *A* and *B*
(with angles of inclination α and β[8]) to the right of *O* and to object
points *C* and *D* (with angles of inclination γ and δ) to the left of *O*
(Fig. 16).[9] We can feel assured that their respective images will
retain this arrangement on the retina. And this is all the clues the
organism needs. Except for the inversion, a consequence of the working of the laws of optics, a consequence of the crossing of the visual
rays in the pupil, the spatial relations of the objects to each other are
mirrored in the distribution of their images on the retina. The actual
distribution depends, of course, also on the position of the sensing
eye. The laws of perspective are laws of image distribution *for a
given point of view.* Perspective does not deal with distribution of
objects in "absolute" space, whatever that word may mean. For the
distribution of the retinal images of points *A, B, O, C, D* to be as indicated in our present example, the pupil (the pole) of the eye must be
at some point P_0. Should the eye, the pupil, change position to any
location P_x in the space that contains the object points *A, B, O, C, D*,
the distribution of their images on the retina would be entirely different. Our diagram makes this clear without any further explanation.

We must now make another assumption. There is sufficient
neuroanatomical and neurophysiological evidence to let us make it
with some assurance. We assume that discrete light stimuli as they
fall upon discrete retinal locations trigger processes of excitation in
these locations which, through ordered and discrete channels (we call
it the optic radiation), finally reach the visual cortex of the brain.[10]
We shall, in other words, assume that the retinal image is *templated*

upon the visual cortex, and that the orderly relationship between discrete stimuli is maintained throughout. We can therefore actually speak of a brain image, which is a homologue of the retinal image, and, at least in a figurative sense, we can speak of a "retina" in the brain. How the organism can best use the information templated *first* from objects upon the retina, *then* from the retina through connecting nerve tracts upon the brain, and *finally* from the brain retina upon the motor executors that are to "handle" the information — that is the question we want to analyze now.

Imagine the simplest of all possible arrangements for visual orientation in the surround: *one* eye in the center of the forehead and forward turned, the way the Cyclopses, those giant monsters of Greek mythology, were said to have carried their single eye. Assume that such a Cyclops' eye is turned on a manifold of details in its field of vision, on a manifold A, B, O, C, D (Fig. 17). The images of these object details will be cast ("templated") on points D, C, O, B, A respectively, of the retina of this eye, in inverted order but with the order preserved. Finally, assume that this order remains unchanged while the stimulus processes from these retinal points ascend toward some higher organization center, the cortex, where (a) these "sensory" (= afferent = centripetal) processes are being "consummated" (= turned into vision) and (b) the appropriate decisions are made as to how to handle the information received. However, since the retinal image is inverted, the stimulus process from, say, object point A at the extreme right end of the visual field will arrive through retinal point A at point A in the extreme left periphery of this cerebral organization center. Obviously, decisions involving object A will be easiest sent, quickest executed, and with least interference, if the pertinent motor (= efferent = centrifugal) impulses are initiated in the left half of our Cyclops' brain and, during their descent toward the executor muscles on the right side of the body, somehow, somewhere, *cross* the midline. However, the inversion of the retinal image also involves the vertical direction. (The retinal image is *not* a "mirror" image but an inverted image). Thus, actions involving some object AA (not shown) to the *right* and also *above* eye level will have to be handled through motor pathways originating in *left* but also *lower* parts of the organization center. (It seems that that little imaginary mannikin, the decision maker in our Cyclops' brain, not only instituted himself on the "wrong" side; he also stands on his head.)

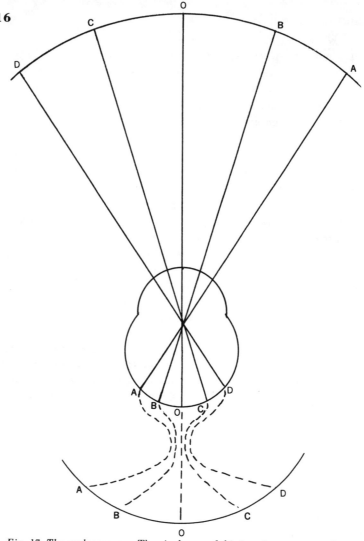

Fig. 17. The cyclopean eye. The single eye of this imaginary creature has a visual field *A* to *D*. The visual impressions cover the retinal area *A* to *D*, in an inverted manner. Except for the inversion (and the reduction of three to two dimensions, not discussed here) the spatial order and arrangement of the retinal image details *A* to *D* match the spatial order and arrangement of the object details *A* to *D* in visible space. The fovea in the center of the retina, at *O*, is covered by the image of point *O* straight ahead. Assume that the retinal images from *A* to *D*, are via nervous connections, templated in an orderly manner upon the visual cortex. Then the brain receives a cyclopean image *A* to *D* which is also inverted. Stimulus impressions from, say, *A*, a point at the extreme right end of the visible world, reach the visual brain at *A* on the extreme left. The spatial order and arrangement of details in the visual brain correspond (except for the inversion) with the spatial order and arrangement of details in the visible world.

It does not really matter that no creature with a cyclopean camera eye is known to exist. Our mental exercise in analyzing this purely imaginary arrangement will still turn out to lead to some quite valid conclusions. We are all Cyclopses if we cover one of our eyes. Even if not as effectively as with two eyes, visual situations can quite well be handled with only one eye. Thus, before we turn to the problem of seeing with two eyes, we are justified in discussing one more aspect of cyclopean vision, the significance of the point O in visible space and of its retinal representation at O.

Let us, then, further assume for a moment that (a) the eye of our Cyclops is motionless relative to his head, and (b) it has a kind of miniature supersensor, a fovea, built in at O in the center of the retina opposite the pupil. The image of an object falling upon this point O would in this case inform our Cyclops that the corresponding object O is *straight ahead*. At the same time O would also be the *best-seen* object. All other points, such as A and B or C and D, would naturally arrange themselves around O, to the right or to the left of this point, the best-seen object, the point of forward *orientation*. Our Cyclops would in fact find that most of his problems of directional visual localization (but only of *directional* visual localization)[11] are solved for him by his single eye.

However, let us not range too far from the set purpose of this discussion. Even if a cyclopean eye were quite an effective tool of spatial orientation, the fact is that no vertebrate is known to exist or ever to have existed with a simple cyclopean eye. Obviously, the visual field of one eye is not sufficient for survival. All vertebrates have two eyes to fathom a much fuller expanse of their ambiance. In fact, many species of fish or bird can, with two eyes placed far laterally, cover almost all of their surround (Fig. 18). They have what Cajal called "panoramic" vision: the right eye covers the right half of their visual world and the left eye the left. (Whether or not there is any part of it binocularly covered Cajal left undetermined in his further studies. So does my diagram. It is irrelevant at the moment.)

The binocular panoramic arrangement added much to the ability of animals so equipped to explore their surround. Nevertheless, it also offered a challenge. Let us analyze both the arrangement and the challenge. We shall do this following Cajal's lead.[12]

Cajal's sketch (Fig. 19a) and a modification of it (Fig. 19b) taken from Linksz (1952) depict another imaginary case, one that, like the cyclopean eye, has as yet been encountered nowhere and never. Both diagrams show the inverted retinal image of the right and left

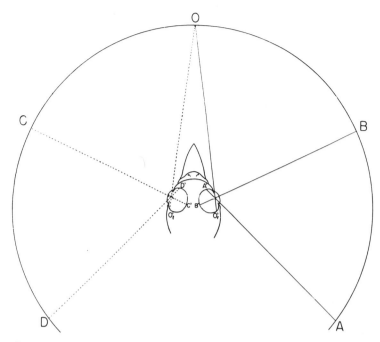

Fig. 18. The binocular "panoramic" arrangement. The right half of the visible world from *A* to *O* covers the retina of the right eye (the image is inverted). The left half of the visible world from *O* to *D* covers the retina of the left eye (also in an inverted manner). The two halves meet at point *O*, the point of orientation, a point seen with both eyes as straight in front, and (if the eyes do not move) at a certain definite distance in front.

half of the visual world, respectively, in the right and left eye of some lower vertebrate (in my diagram it is clearly a bird) with panoramic vision. The retinal images are shown projected via neural connections, and under preservation of their spatial order, upon corresponding lobes of the brain: the right eye's image upon the right brain and the left eye's image upon the left brain. As I said, this arrangement has never actually been met with. Simple as it may seem, like the cyclopean eye, Nature must have found it an impossible arrangement, one unable to serve its biologic purposes. The lack of utility of such an arrangement is, I confess, much more dramatically presented in Cajal's rather primitive sketch (Fig. 19*a*) than in my much more detailed diagram (Fig. 19*b*). The *L* in Cajal's sketch stands for

Lobus opticus, the structure in the lower vertebrate's brain upon which the optic radiations project.) Still, in some respects my more naturalistic diagram, a horizontal cross section through a bird's head and eyes, has some merit. It shows in greater detail some of the consequences the arrangement would have. Take the points A'' and D'', the "cerebral" representations of the retinal points A' and D': they would be thrown into loci of undue proximity, while in the reality of the surrounding object world the corresponding points A and D are farthest apart. But even worse is the confusion that would befall point O, the point straight ahead and also at a rather well-defined distance from our paradigm's eyes (cf. Fig. 18). This important point, on which a creature like the bird depicted would quite naturally orient itself (hence the label O given this point), would be represented twice — in brain loci that are far apart and in different brain hemispheres. Moreover, since it is impossible for objects and eye images to be completely motionless, the representation of this object point O would oscillate from one hemisphere to the other. If we postulate that preservation of spatial order in the retinal images and in their projection upon the visual cortex is the basis of meaningful and purposeful space perception, then we must admit that an arrangement such as the one we are now envisaging would serve space perception poorly. It would certainly make effective handling of visual messages difficult if not impossible, and effective handling of the visible world, of objects in the ambiance, is the sole biologic purpose of vision. In fact, this arrangement involving *two* eyes would be much inferior to a cyclopean arrangement which, although not of sufficient efficiency, would at least not suffer from intrinsic contradictions.

Thus Cajal realized that orderly and organized perception of spatial relations cannot be achieved if the retinal images, inverted as they are, are projected upon the brain in the manner just depicted. We may add that nowhere has there been found even an indication that Nature made an attempt at reinversion of inverted retinal images (which Descartes suggested and which, in fact, would eliminate the contradiction). It was a true stroke of genius when Cajal realized that this whole dilemma resolved itself in the simplest manner if the *optic nerves cross*, as in fact they do. This can readily be seen in Cajal's second sketch (Fig. 20a), and in my more naturalistic modification of it (Fig. 20b), in which the rearrangement is shown in greater detail.

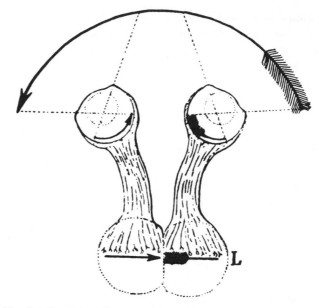

Fig. 19a. Cajal's original diagram of the imaginary case in which the optic nerves do not cross.

Almost as if by magic, everything falls into its appropriate place: separateness and proximalness of individual object details, centralness and peripheralness in the field of vision — all are correctly duplicated on the "brain retina." For all practical purposes of visual orientation, the total *binocularly provided* brain image becomes a faithful replica, a map or template, except for the inversion, of the object world. The two eyes with their enlarged visual field (and in spite of it) furnish a brain image with which handling the surround is not at all impossible. Take the object points A and D, widely separated in the object world and represented by the image points A'' and D'' in the brain, with the retinal loci A' and D' serving as go-betweens. Thanks, so to speak, to the crossing of the optic nerves, the position of A'' and D'' relative to each other now corresponds to what we like to call reality. The same can be said about the relative positions of points B'' and C'', the representations, respectively, of object points B and C. Finally, the same can be said about the orientation point O in front of the animal (Fig. 19*b*), where right and left visual field meet. This point O forms two retinal images, one in each

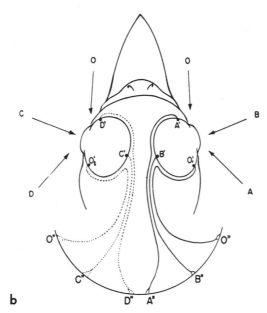

Fig. 19b. Horizontal cross section through the eyes and the visual "cortex" of a bird with panoramic vision; the imaginary case where there is no decussation of optic nerves. The diagram is a modification of Cajal's. Both Cajal's diagram and this one indicate how each eye maintains for itself as much as it can of the spatial order of one-half of the external manifold. As in Fig. 18, the images in the right eye duplicate the spatial order from *A* to *O*, and those in the left eye the spatial order from *O* to *D*. But if each retina were projected upon the higher visual center of its own side, the two halves would cease to be continuations of each other and the total spatial order within the brain would finally be destroyed. Cajal was certainly correct to stress the fact that such a neuroanatomic situation would be biologically impossible. In fact, it never occurs.

eye, and the two images together furnish some kind of a redoubled, reinforced brain image (Fig. 20*b*). In Fig. 20*b*, the two images are shown next to each other; in the physical reality of the visual brain they must coincide. It would be incompatible with the biologic purpose of vision for the brain to fashion *two* cortical images of *one* object of the surround, one through each eye. In fact, here we meet a new phenomenon which we call "fusion," with one object forming two retinal images but producing a single, quasi-amalgamated visual impression. It is a new kind of vision: single vision binocularly mediated. (This remarkable faculty, binocular single vision, in the case depicted in Fig. 20*b* must be limited to a small common area of the

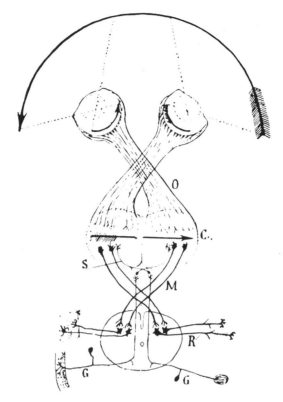

Fig. 20a. Cajal's original diagram of a case in which the optic nerves cross. The diagram also indicates the crossing of the motor pathways, *M*, and of the sensory pathways, *S*.

total visual field and will, at the moment, not be considered further.)

We see, then, that in animals with panoramic vision (in animals which cover the right half of their visual world with the right eye and the left half with the other eye) total crossing of the optic nerves is the *sine qua non* of the preservation of spatial order in the visual brain, even if the order is preserved in an inverted manner.[13] Though our diagrams cannot indicate this well, the inversion also holds for the vertical aspect of the field of vision. Objects that are in the *lower* half of the animal's visible world imprint upon the *upper* (coronal) quadrants of the visual cortex, while the visual impressions from the *upper* half of the visible world cover the *lower* (caudal) brain areas. Ultimately, the total brain image is inverted in the sense of both right

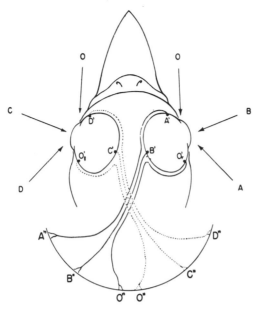

Fig. 20b. Horizontal cross section through the eyes and the visual "cortex" of a bird with panoramic vision, the case in which there is total crossing of optic nerves. Each eye separately retains a replica of the spatial order of one-half of the external manifold in the spatial order of its own retinal images. Images in the right eye mirror the spatial order of the right half of the visible world; images in the left eye mirror the spatial order of the left half of the visible world. But only through total crossing of the optic nerves can a replica of the spatial order of the *total* external manifold be templated upon the receiving brain. Total crossing makes it possible that, to some external order *ABOCD*, an order *A″B″O″C″D″* finally becomes coordinated in the bird's brain.

and left and top and bottom. With all this complexity the brain image is truly cyclopean: *two eyes looking in two different directions together map or template a cyclopean impression, consistent with "reality," upon the visual brain!*[14] Which brings us to our main point of interest: the nerve tracts that carry motor impulses to skeletal muscles. They arrange themselves in a parallel manner. *The motor impulses to the extremities of either side of the body originate from* (or, more accurately, can be traced to) *the opposite brain hemisphere.* As Cajal expressed it, visual impressions from the left side of the panorama converge on centers in the right brain and motor messages to the left extremities diverge from centers that are also in the right brain. Obviously, to reach their destination from right brain to left extremities, the motor tracts (the efferent or centrifugal nerve tracts) must cross the midline. By now, everyone knows about this most conspicuous feature in the organization of our neuroanatomy, the so-called "pyramidal crossing." It *exists*, like the crossing of the optic nerves. Cajal did not have to imagine it.

But the parallelism between the optical and motor arrangement is even more striking: not only do the motor fibers cross; their distribution also follows (is also adjusted for) the inversion of the retinal image and the brain image. In their downward course from the motor areas of the brain, the more caudally originating motor fibers leave the central nervous system first; they are destined for the head, neck, and upper extremities. The more coronally originating motor fibers, destined for the lower extremities, continue their descent within the spinal cord and leave it at appropriately lower, more caudal levels. Our little mannikin decision maker resides on the wrong side and stands on his head. The motor arrangements are strictly cyclopean.

As we can also see from Cajal's diagram, the pattern set by the motor pathways is reduplicated once more in the arrangement of the sensory, the proprioceptive nerve structures. We see in Cajal's figure two additional neurons rather primitively indicated: their bipolar cell body earmarks them as sensory (afferent or centripetal) neurons. They are shown originating on some effector structures, one on a muscle fiber, the other on some unidentifiable sensory end organ. (Note the fibers marked *G*.) They are turning upward in the diagram, toward another crossing, the so-called sensory decussation. Their job is to bring the message of accomplishment or failure back to the locus of impulse origination. (Our current technical term "sensory feedback" was not known in Cajal's times.) They must cross the midline to be able to do this. Moreover, they too comply with the upside-down — more accurately, "inverted" — arrangement of the retinal images, with the mapping of the retinal images in the visual brain, and with the efferent innervation template. Nature must have had very good biologic reasons, must have seen very great biologic gain in this arrangement, since she has taken the pains to build such complex and complicated structures. As Dr. Einstein said, speaking about the wisdom of Nature: "God does not play dice."

In reality, this seemingly complex arrangement is the simplest possible arrangement. It satisfies an important principle of structuring in the nervous system, to which the name "neurobiotaxis" was

given by the Dutch neuroanatomist Ariens Kappers (1921). According
to this principle, *related functions localize in adjacent structures*.
Messages have to be processed. Information must be handled. Handling must be quick and effective. The animal sees for a purpose; it
does not have the time or the means to contemplate. For a message
conveyed through the visual apparatus to become most useful, best
usable, the motor executor has to be reached through the smallest
number of relays, via the shortest route, with as little interference as
possible. As visual impressions from the animal's left surround converge upon the right half of its brain, it is certainly in keeping with
purposeful functioning that motor impulses toward the left half of the
body diverge from the right half of the brain and that feedback information from the left half of the body converges back onto it.

The kind of vision we have just discussed (Cajal's "panoramic"
arrangement) was partially superseded in higher animals, including
Man, by the gradual overlapping of the visual fields. Eyes are in more
lateral positions of the skull in "lower" vertebrates. They moved into
more and more forward positions in the more "advanced" species.
Goethe had already surmised (1784) some such happening in his ex-
tended comparative anatomy studies of the intermaxillary bone, a
bony facial structure that gets more and more rudimentary the
"higher" the vertebrate species. Goethe saw in this fact a hint of the
possibility of evolution (he used the term "metamorphosis") quite a
few years before Darwin first publicly dared to doubt the immuta-
bility of species since Creation. Because of this feature of evolution,
because of the forward drift of the eyeballs, a significant part of the
visual field (in Man some 110 degrees of it) covers both eyes and both
halves of the brain retina. There still exists, however, a considerable
expanse of, say, the right visual field that is covered *only* by the right
eye and through the right eye only by the left brain.

Binocular overlap necessitated a rearrangement of connections
from eyes to brain. Figure 21 will help visualize Nature's answer to
this new challenge (see page 229). It is the feature of half-crossing of
the optic nerves. Nature rescued, so to speak, the strictly cyclopean
templating of visible space on the brain retina (an arrangement without which ordered motor reaction to visual messages is impossible)
in spite of binocularity. (Or perhaps I should say while at the same
time rising to the opportunity of binocular coverage.) Thus, whether
panoramic arrangement or binocular fusional arrangement, the right

half of the visual world is imaged, mapped, templated in the left brain and *only* in the left brain. Indeed, if we compare Figs. 17, 20b and 21, we must be struck by the essential similarity.

The brain retina has remained cyclopean whatever the other arrangements. And as far as the motor and the sensory tracts to and from the skeletal musculature are concerned, their distribution, too, remains *entirely* cyclopean. The arrangements in the motor cortex represent a template of the cyclopean brain retina in the primate no less than in the lower vertebrate. *The feature of binocularity is totally ignored!* The pyramidal (motor) tracts to the skeletal muscles cross completely on Man as they do in the lower vertebrate, and the proprioceptive (sensory or feedback) pathways after crossing the midline converge in a region that again is nothing but a template of the motor arrangement. The centrifugal (motor) neurons originate from the precentral (pre-Rolandic) convolution of the "wrong" side, the neurons to the lower extremities from more coronal aspects, the neurons to the upper extremities from more caudal parts. The centripetal (proprioceptive) neurons reach the postcentral (post-Rolandic) convolution in an appropriate manner. The structural principle of "templating the template of a template" could not be more rigorously observed.

We have, then, finally arrived at at least one answer: *The pyramidal tracts of all vertebrates cross because their retinal images are inverted and* (this is an addition to Cajal's statement) *because the brain retina is cyclopean.* This answer holds for Man just as much as for the lower vertebrates that Cajal analyzed. Thus, the matrix behind the right hand's skills *must* be the left brain. Whatever the circumstances that made our right hand dominant, we are leftbrained as a consequence. There is nothing in the original basic anatomy of the vertebrate brain that makes the left brain dominant, although there are some indications that by now the left brain, the "speech area" in Man's left brain, is *ab ovo* destined to be dominant. At least the bulk of the temporal lobe on the left side (it houses most of our nonvisual language equipment) is significantly greater than the bulk of the same lobe on the other side (Geschwind, 1972). In the final analysis, Man is leftbrained because his heart is on the left side and my seemingly witty remark turns out to be serious: "We write with the right hand because our heart is on the left side." But it is not at all impossible for the right brain to take over. Even a "speech center" can develop in the right brain secondarily if damage to the one in the left brain has occurred early enough in life. The anatomical basis is provided. It is just never used in most of us. The same holds, of course, for lefthandedness, especially lefthandedness in writing. The anatomical basis for all the skills of the left hand is there, in the right brain. If heredity or circumstances favor *its* dominance, there is no reason why these skills cannot develop.[15] We just have to think of the ambidextrous performance of the pianist or the surgeon to be impressed by the capabilities of the left hand. And Professor Kolisch, the "lefthanded" violinist is certainly a shining example of what "training" can accomplish. He trained himself to bow the violin with the left hand though he surely was (and still is) leftbrained. I cannot believe that such a great sin against an apparently lefthanded child's personality is being committed if we try to train his right hand for writing. The chances that as far as speech is concerned he is leftbrained are overwhelming anyway.

NOTES

[1]Our speech "center" (which is what more than anything else makes us humans human) is, in the overwhelming majority of us (lefthanders included), in the left brain (Goodglass and Quadfasel, 1954).

[2]The crossing of motor nerve fibers (of the fibers carrying the bulk of impulses that contract our muscles, e.g., that move a limb) over the midline occurs in the part of the brain that connects it to the spinal chord. The old anatomists fancied that this particular structure resembles a pyramid. Hence we use the term *pyramidal* tract or tracts when we want to identify these crossing, or crossed, motor tracts. They mainly carry impulses from what we call the motor areas of the brain *out* of the central nervous system, toward our motor appliances, the muscles. They are therefore also identified as *efferent* (nerves or tracts). In contradistinction, *sensory* tracts carry messages, information, about these appliances and also information on the surrounding world *into* the central nervous system. They are therefore also referred to as *afferent* (nerves or tracts). To be more specific, the impulses to, say, the muscles of the limbs "originate" (can be traced) from brain areas that are *in front of* one of the brain's main dividers, the central or Rolandian groove. Hence the term precentral or pre-Rolandic brain areas. (There are two of them, one on the right side, one on the left.) The information about the status or performance of these muscles, runs (can be traced, is fed back) toward so-called sensory areas behind that divider. Hence these sensory areas are also called postcentral or post-Rolandic. The information about the surrounding world (e.g., information carried by light from visible objects into our eyes or by sound toward

our ears) runs toward other brain areas, specialized for the reception of such information messages. Only the sensory areas specialized for the information received through the eyes, the so-called visual area of the brain located at the posterior pole of the brain hemispheres, will be of interest in this exposition.

[3]"Coronal" means near the crown and refers to structures in upper, more forward aspects of the brain: "caudal" means near the tail and refers to structures that are further down.

[4]There are twelve nerve pairs that originate from or feed into the brain itself. They are called the cranial nerves. All other neural messages (e.g., those to and from the limbs) leave or enter via the spinal chord.

[5]Visible space is a cover word for all the objects in the surround from which light rays can reach the inside of the eyes, the retina. My chair is in my subjective space (I feel its seat pressing against my seat), but it is not at the moment within my visible space. The walls of my room limit this space. The horizon limits it. The sky limits it. Visible space is "limited" space.

[6]A coordinate system is a set of magnitudes used to describe the position of geometric elements, e.g., points, in space. Different coordinate systems exist. Descartes' system, the so-called Cartesian coordinate system, is the best known. Our purposes will be best served by a system of so-called polar coordinates. Such a system includes a pole (a point of origin), a polar axis (a line through the pole) to which is ascribed zero inclination, and radius vectors or vectors (other lines through the pole) whose the inclination to the polar axis is measured and expressed in some numerical terms, say degrees. To describe the position of some point P in the space of polar coordinates, one measures its distance from the pole along the vector that connects the two (the point and the pole) and specifies the vector by its angle (or angles) of inclination.

[7]Although rays as such are purely constructions of the mind, in our description we are not too far from reality. We can imagine that our visual rays are the trajectories of light particles (they are called photons) traveling from the objects through the pupil up to the retina, where they become involved in the formation of the retinal image.

[8]The angles are not indicated in order to leave the diagram uncluttered.

[9]This is a somewhat simplified presentation. It refers to only one angle, the angle of inclination in the plane of the diagram (assumed to be horizontal). It also neglects the distance factor, the distance of the seen objects O, A, B, etc., from the sensing eye. If the position of a point in the space of polar coordinates is to be accurately characterized, two angles and a vector quantity are needed. (I cannot deal with these aspects of space perception in this context.)

[10]The limited surface area of the brain toward which the visual excitations are channeled.

[11]There is one clue which the cyclopean eye cannot offer. Take, e.g., the point B on the radius vector P_oB of the coordinate system of this eye (Fig. 16). You can push the object point B farther or nearer along this vector, yet its image will still always fall on point B of the retina. As the eighteenth-century philosopher Bishop Berkeley clearly noted, the single eye cannot furnish any reliable information regarding the actual distance of any object point from the "fund of the eye." We also cannot have true stereoscopic vision with only one eye. All a single eye can offer is reliable information about

direction, "directional visual localization." (See my book *Physiology of the Eye: Volume II, Vision*, 1952.)

[12]Cajal's original ideas on the subject were first published in 1898 in Spanish. Later he incorporated them into the French edition of his classic neuroanatomy (1911). The same material also exists as a small monograph (1899) in German. Neither of these publications is easily accessible. Reproductions of two of Cajal's original diagrams, with comments, are to be found in Linksz (1952). They are also reproduced here as Figs. 19*a* and 20*a*. The interested reader will find Cajal's views, and much of the material presented in this appendix, discussed in the book of that great encyclopedist, the late Professor Gordon Walls, *The Vertebrate Eye* (1963). My indebtedness to this book — a source book if there ever was one — cannot be sufficiently stressed, even if it is not specifically mentioned in all the appropriate places.

[13]It should be mentioned in passing that B and C are objects on the optical axis of the right and the left eye respectively. Both of them project their image upon *a* fovea, B' in the right eye, C' in the left. I say *a* fovea and not *the* fovea for a good reason: the depicted bird has two foveas in each eye — the points on which the images of O fall are *also* foveas, i.e., areas specially endowed for a special task. Theoretically, a bird can keep its head still and see three objects in detail at the same time, which is much more than we can do. The foveas B' and C' are usually referred to as nasal foveas: O'_l and O'_r are called temporal foveas.

[14]The insight of the ancient Greeks into the working of Nature was truly uncanny. Edith Hamilton in her classic *Greek Mythology* retells the story of the Cyclops Polyphemus, the evil giant whom Ulysses finally blinded. Miss Hamilton "quotes" a dialogue between Galathea (with whom our monster was in love) and her sister Doris, a discussion in which Galathea assures her sister that in spite of having only one eye Polyphemus sees as well as if he had two. The idea that one sees better with two eyes than he can with one must have been understood by the Greeks. Why otherwise mention the exception? It should be interesting to note in this connection that the Hebrew will never use the plural when referring to the "evil eye." Otherwise the Bible almost always refers to "eyes." I can still hear my father reciting his favorite psalm (121) before we went to bed:

I will lift up mine eyes unto the hills,

[15]I have several patients who are left handed and have a history of injury to the right arm, or right shoulder, at birth or in early childhood. I have no proof that they are not genuine lefthanders, but the chances are that they are not.

On Ocular Asymmetry — On Ocular Dominance

To my mind, we have arrived at some quite satisfactory answers to the questions posed at the beginning of Appendix A. We should now be ready to turn to a related problem, ocular asymmetry and ocular dominance. Figure 21 will be helpful as an introduction. The figure indicates, rather schematically, the binocular visual field of the primate Man. It extends from *B* to *C* and includes a point we have been calling *O* in the cyclopean and panoramic arrangements. In Man the point *O* is a point of much less distinction. Though I have retained the letter as a reminder of its old significance, in Man this point is not the pivotal point of orientation any longer. It does not serve egocentric (falsely called "absolute") localization. Even if the head is held straight, *O* does not serve as a clue to the direction straight ahead. It merely denotes the point of *momentary* binocular foveal fixation (hence the two foveas are also marked *O*). It is *momentarily* the "best seen" point and the point at which the left and right half of our panorama *momentarily* meet.[1] It is ocular mobility that has changed all this. Our eyes having become mobile, our foveas, *O* and *O*,[2] can now explore ("best see") any point in visible space toward which the extraocular muscles will carry the eyes. That in my diagram point *O* is still on the midline of symmetry merely serves the esthetics of the picture. (The imaginary triangle one can construct through *O* and the two foveas is an isosceles in the diagram; it would have no such shape were *O* displaced right or left.)

As the figure indicates, the binocularly seen *left* field portion, *O* to *C*, covers the *total* available *temporal* retinal territory, *O* to *C*, in the right eye. These messages reach the right visual cortex. The pertinent nerve fibers remain uncrossed. The binocularly seen *right* field portion, *O* to *B*, covers *part* of the available *nasal* retinal territory, *O* to *B* of the same eye, but *not all* of the available territory. Another part of the nasal retinal territory, from *B* to *A*, is covered by the right *monocular* temporal visual field (in clinical parlance we refer to it as the "temporal crescent" of the visual field), from *B* to *A*. There is *more* retinal territory nasally from the foveas than temporally. The foveas are not in the middle. And from this asymmetry it follows that the share of the right eye in covering the right field of activity (the "aggression" field as I have called it) is greater than its share in covering the left field of activity. *All* the messages from the nasal retina of the right eye reach the left brain. Thus, the coverage of the right field of activity by the *left* brain via the *right* eye is wider, more extensive (we can assume it is more significant) than the share of the *right* brain in the coverage of the *left* field of activity, also via the *right* eye. In other words, in spite of binocularity the *right eye covers more right visual field than left visual field* and covers some right visual field exclusively. Its stake in the right field is predominant. And whatever reduplicating coverage of a part of the *right* field of activity the *left* eye brings to the *left* cortex (via uncrossed optic nerve fibers), this coverage is less in bulk and, we can assume, less in significance. Furthermore, the temporal half-retina of each eye is "hooked up" to the brain by a phylogenetically younger arrangement: the optic nerve fibers from the temporal retinal halves do *not* cross. All in all, the *temporal* retinal halves are the less significant information carriers, obviously the nondomineering halves. In contradistinction, the *nasal* retinal halves carry on with the phylogenetically older "panoramic" tradition: *each* covers one half of the *total* available visual field *and* their fibers cross. They could therefore also be called the primordial halves, the "panoramic" halves, and, obviously, they are the domineering halves. In the final arrangement, the stake of, say, the *left brain* in the *right visual field* is absolute: *all* messages from the right half of the visual field (*some* through the left eye, *most* through the right eye) reach the left brain, and only the left brain. In this respect, there is no difference between fish, bird, and Man. (We seem to be so much intrigued by the mysteries of binocular coverage that often we are not even aware of this essential fact.) Strange as it may sound at first, the brain retina does not even need the "tem-

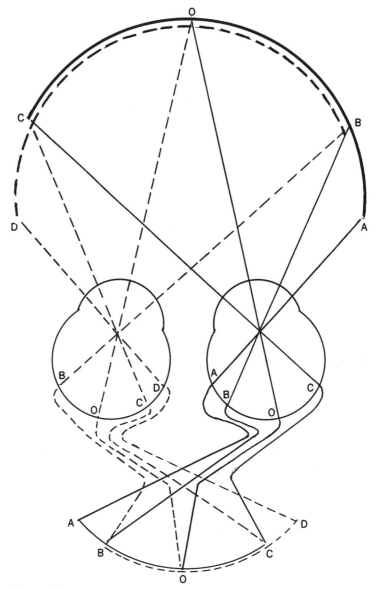

Fig. 21. The physical basis of binocular (human) vision. The visual fields of the right eye (———) and the left eye (— — —) partially overlap. The foveal lines of gaze (right O———O, left O— — —O) meet in a point O, the best seen point. Each retina consists of a nasal (medial) and a temporal (lateral) half which meet at O, the best see-

ing point. Each nasal half retina covers the *total* field of its own side. Thus, O to A in the right retina covers the *whole* right half of the visual field from O to A. The temporal half retina is a smaller half. Thus, the temporal "half" retina of the right eye from O to C covers only *part* of the left visual field, from O to C. *All* stimulus impressions from the right visual field, O to A, are templated on the left visual brain, O to A, via the nasal half retina, A to O, of the right eye. However, part of the right visual field, from O to B, sends a second, reinforcing message via the temporal retina of the left eye, O to B, toward the same, the left, visual brain. In other words, the portion O to B of the right visual field and the region O to B in the left visual brain are covered twice. Nevertheless, the arrangement of impressions in the visual brain is strictly cyclopean. The visual field extends from the extreme right point A to the extreme left point D. Although in an inverted manner, the distribution A, B, O, C, D of the visual field is duplicated in the visual brain.

poral" retinal contributions to receive full visual field coverage. If the temporal retinas were both blind (this happens in binasal hemianopia), the cyclopean arrangement in our brain retina would still be complete. (Blot out, in Fig. 21, the contributions from the two temporal half-retinas. The full cyclopean coverage of the brain retina will be there just the same.[3]) But we would have no binocular vision. Our temporal half-retinas are grafted, so to speak, upon our basically cyclopean visual brain without distorting the cyclopean arrangement in the least. The "temporal" contribution adds the binocularity feature — new, gratifying, but like red-green vision *not essential*.

The diagram, by the way, also reveals that our foveas are placed at a strategic position: where our nasal ("panoramic") and our temporal ("binocularity providing") retinal halves meet. They carry on with one tradition of the "nasal" foveas of the bird of prey ("best vision"). They cannot fulfill the job of the bird's "temporal" foveas. Obviously, human vision is concerned with three items: exploration (mobility), detail (foveas), and, last and least, stereopsis (binocularity). Visual orientation, egocentric localization, distance perception are shortchanged in the transaction. We see space more through our memories, our past experiences. *We see space more with our brain than with our eyes.* We think we "see" the distance of objects. In reality, we mostly "judge" it. (See Note 13, p. 229.)

There is no need to continue this line of thought in all its details with respect to the left eye. The fact is that the dominant left brain (whatever the reason or reasons for its dominance) receives a greater quantity of information about the dominant right activity field (whatever the reason or reasons for its dominance) through the crossed fibers (the more ancient arrangement) from the right eye than through the uncrossed fibers (the more recent arrangement) from the left eye. Or to put it differently: the right hand's action field is *primarily* covered by the right eye and the left brain. The visual feedback control of most of the activities of the *right* hand occurs primarily via right-eye-to-left-brain, to a lesser degree via left-eye-to-left-brain and only rarely (the right hand must have crossed the visual midline) through the right brain. This makes the right eye the major shareholder in the right field-right hand-left brain dominance combine. The fact that our visual panorama consists of a right half field (covered by the left brain) and a left half field (covered symmetrically by the right brain) does not prima facie exclude the possibility that one-half of the visual field somehow exceeds the other half in significance. Similarly, the fact that we have binocular vision, and especially that we ordinarily fixate with both eyes, does not prima facie exclude the possibility that, while simultaneously engaged in the business of binocular vision, one eye may, in a sense, be the leading eye.

However, there are some questions to be answered, some objections to be hurdled. Hand dominance and brain dominance are clearly interrelated. Apparently we cannot account for a concept of eye dominance with the same assuredness.

One objection is obvious to begin with. Retinal asymmetry is a bilateral, a symmetrical feature, and the right visual cortex also receives unequal loads of information via the two eyes, more via the crossed fibers from the left eye and less via the noncrossing fibers from the right eye. But this objection is easily dismissed. Ocular dominance (whatever this term may imply) cannot be explained by eye anatomy just as hand dominance cannot be explained by brain anatomy. There is no *gross* anatomical arrangement in the eyes themselves or in their brain connections that could account for the dominance of, say, the right eye. But there is also nothing in the gross anatomy of the right hand or in the gross structure of the left brain to make it dominant. One hand is the mirror image of the other. And the pre-Rolandic (motor) area in one hemisphere is the mirror image of that in the other hemisphere. There are also no anatomically identifiable "centers" for speech, for reading, in just one hemisphere and not in the other. Potentially, either hand can be dominant and either hemisphere could be leading, even the harborer of the language faculties although some chromosomal preferential "memory" must by now have established itself. Such memory will favor, even facilitate, the dominance of the right hand and of the left brain and the institution of what comes nearest to a "language center" in the left hemisphere, unless some event, inclement and incidental, prevents this.[4] Potentially, then, either eye could be dominant. It is the right hand's dominance (if I may once more voice this opinion) that made and still makes the left brain the dominant brain half *secondarily*. Dominance of the right eye (its statistically more common occurrence in the righthanded and left-brained population) is at best a *tertiary* affair, some very late acquisition easily uncoupled.

But there are certain even more deeply rooted conceptual difficulties that make it hard to accept ocular dominance as an entity. There is some reason for serious doubt. Perhaps there is no such thing as ocular dominance? One cannot simply parallel ocular dominance with hand dominance or brain dominance. There exists a strict vectorial (neuroanatomic) relationship between, say, left brain and right hand. If one is (or has become) dominant, then the dominant character of the other is quasi-anatomically foreordained. (It makes no difference, so to speak, which is the chicken and which is the egg.) Righthandedness must make the left brain the matrix of its skills because the motor tracts cross. Leftbrainedness (if one assumes that by now there is some inborn, chromosomal, even anatomic, predestination) must make the right hand dominant for the very same reason.

No such straight anatomic relationship exists between the oculomotor arrangements of, say, the left brain and the right eye. The law of neurobiotaxis and the template principle (both discussed earlier), both require some "rewiring" in the oculorotary arrangements of the primate. In the primate the temporal retina of, say, the left eye is templated upon the left visual brain (via fibers uncrossed. But it is templated upon *an already preexisting* map, upon the basic, phylogenetically much older, "panoramic" template mapped upon the left visual cortex via the nasal retina of the right eye. The oculorotary rewiring follows this new arrangement as accurately as the pyramidal crossing follows the inverted brain image. *Bilateral oculoperceptual coverage templates bilateral oculorotary coverage.* Thus, the left oculorotary "centers" (impulse originators would be a better term) send impulses to some oculorotary muscles of the right eye and also to appropriate oculorotary muscles of the left eye. They follow a new law, Hering's law, which expresses this fact in violation, so to speak, of what we would call the old, established "pyramidal" law which, let me emphasize again, remains inviolate with respect to *all* other bodily motor innervation modalities. The anatomy of the motor arrangements from brain to eyes is truly unique. In any event, that unequivocal relationship which in the majority of us makes the dominant left brain *and* the dominant right hand an anatomically foreordained *dominance unit,* that unequivocal relationship does not hold for, say, left brain and right eye. Here is the difficulty that the concept of ocular dominance must surmount. We *can* ask the question: "Perhaps there is no such thing? Perhaps there cannot be such thing? Perhaps even the concept is spurious?"

Let me once more analyze ocular motor neuroanatomy with a view to this particular problem. But before I do this, let me make a remark pertinent to ocular motility in a more general way: From the time we first began to study anatomy, we became used to thinking of muscles as movers of bulk, of bones or joints. (We even refer to the majority of the muscles innervated by pyramidal tract fibers as "skeletal" muscles.) And we readily apply such a description to the extraocular muscles. However, a certain refinement in our thinking with regard to the eyes is in order. Dextroversion[5] of the eyes, to give an example, is initiated by contraction of the lateral rectus muscle of the right eye to turn the *right* eyeball right and by simultaneous contraction of the medial rectus muscle of the left eye to turn the *left* eyeball right. As clinicians we are used to referring to these two muscles as "yoke"[6] muscles. They rotate both of our eyes to the right *in unison,* under the direction of Hering's law of the equality of impulse. (We have six pairs of such yoke muscles. Nature has obviously taken great pains to safeguard rotation of both eyes in all possible directions *in unison.*)

While the descriptive term "dextroversion" is certainly impeccable (we can actually observe the front of the eyes rolling in unison toward the right) we will achieve deeper insight into the biological purpose of such oculorotation if we keep in mind that what the *right* lateral rectus muscle is actually accomplishing in terms of function is rotating the *right nasal half-retina* to cover the *right* panoramic visual field, while the medial rectus muscle of the *left* eye is rotating the *temporal half-retina* of the *left* eye to double-cover part (but only part!) of the same visual field. A similar rationale holds good, of course, for the antagonist pair of yoke muscles, for the lateral rectus muscle of the left eye and the medial rectus muscle of the right eye. We make a much more meaningful statement if we say that each of the two lateral rectus muscles rotates its respective nasal half-retina (the primordial retinas with their crossing optic nerve fibers) to cover one-half of the total momentary panorama, while each of the two medial rectus muscles rotates its respective temporal half-retina (the "neo-"retinas, we might call them, with their noncrossing optic nerve fibers) to double-cover the binocular part of the half visual field, but *only* the binocular part. This built-in asymmetry cannot leave the oculomotor apparatus unaffected. We have seen that, in spite of the binocularity feature, the retinal input into, say, the left brain is greater via the right eye than via the left eye: the ancient "panoramic" input arrangement remains prevalent. We should not be surprised to find the output arrangements to be a simple template of this particular mode of input. Thus we may expect that *in spite of Hering's law*, the ancient "pyramidal" motor output arrangement (left brain to right eye via crossing motor neurons) remains prevalent nevertheless. These are further instances of that double symmetrical asymmetry that we can encounter in all binocular arrangements, the logical ("natural") sequence of the nasal-temporal asymmetry of each retina. Our right eye always covers more right visual territory than left visual territory, and our right eye always covers more right visual territory than the left eye does.

The "pioneering" into yet unknown reaches of the right field of activity is always done by the right eye. If I said earlier that the right eye is a shareholder in the right field-right hand-left brain dominance combine, then, it seems, neither binocularity nor Hering's law of bilateral innervation can destroy the intimacy of this relationship.

I am a great believer in the symbolism of the body. (It was Goethe's belief that Nature, even if not in words, tries to "let us in" on her plans and schemes.[7]) Thus, if Nature found it worthwhile for each lateral rectus muscle to have its own nucleus (the so-called sixth-nerve nucleus) and its own nerve (the abducens nerve), then this conspicuous circumstance signifies significance. The lateral rectus muscles are, as I have said, rotators of the respective nasal retinas. Rotating each nasal retina to cover its *total* panoramic half-field of vision is, obviously, a prime task. Why otherwise does each lateral rotator muscle have a nucleus of its own, a nerve of its own?[8] And besides, the arrangement is tradition-proved: the nervous connections from oculorotary cort.cal areas to the lateral rectus muscles run the pure, traditional "pyramidal" course. There can be no question about their simple and total crossing. In contradistinction, the medial rectus muscles are rotators of the respective temporal half-retinas, the new halves, the nonpanoramic halves, the noncrossing halves, the binocular-vision-providing halves. Seemingly they don't each deserve a nucleus of their own, each a nerve of their own. Hence the conspicuous asymmetry even in the anatomy of the two innervation systems: one (the sixth-nerve complex) is sharply defined, simply outlined, with the right and left sides clearly separated; the other (the medial rectus muscle-innervating complex) is as yet not even clarified in its morphology. The innervation of the medial rectus muscles is grafted upon an ancient mass (or mess) of cells (the third-nerve double nucleus) in which what belongs to one side or the other, what fiber sequence crosses, does not cross, or even crosses and re-crosses from brain to muscle has not yet been identified with certainty. (The student of neuroanatomy will be aware of the different schemata suggested to unravel the complexities of the third nerve double nucleus.) Clearly, in spite of all the revolutionary new arrangements, the orthodoxy of the old panoramic-pyramidal input-output arrangement prevails over the binocular-vision-providing arrangement. As the arrangement suggests, exploration of the surround, the primordial panoramic function, clearly the more ancient in the Jacksonian hierarchy of functions is a matter that mostly concerns the nasal half-retinas and the respective lateral rectus muscles. Binocular vision, stereopsis, and (as we shall see) convergence are affairs that concern the temporal half-retinas and are governed by our medial rectuses. They are newer, less essential, easily lost, easily missed, often even missing functions. (The disorientation following paralysis of a lateral rectus muscle is known to clinicians. So is the difference in the pathophysiology of exo- and esodeviations, though this is not the occasion to discuss them.)

To return to our present subject, we can, then, state that there is ample anatomical justification for a concept of ocular dominance: there exists a *continuous undercurrent of monocular vision* (panoramic vision) in spite of all the provisions for binocularity. Binocular vision, sensory fusion, motor adjustments for sensory fusion,[9] and Hering's law are all not contradictory to a concept of one eye's dominance. They are all later grafts, later mappings on a basically panoramic-pyramidal setup of eyes and brain. If such a thing as hand dominance can exist in spite of the basically symmetrical nature of hand and brain anatomies, then so can eye dominance in spite of the symmetrical nature of the respective anatomies — in fact, in spite of the truly exceptional circumstance that each brain half, even if to different degrees, stimulates the motor machinery of both eyes. And with the right hand-left brain-right lateral rectus muscle complex firmly entrenched, the right eye must be the unchallenged favorite of choice for the role of being dominant. It is a weak dominance, a late-late acquisition in the Jacksonian hierarchy of functions.

The unique advantage, of course, of, say, a dominant right eye over a dominant right hand is that whatever this right eye does and wherever this right eye turns, it always covers some left visual territory (via the right temporal half-retina) with the right visual brain. In fact, human eyes with their considerable visual field overlap are unique in this regard: whatever our eyes do, one eye always engages *both* sides of the brain[10] and (even if not its totality) the greatest part of the cyclopean brain retina.[11] This keeps the motor mechanisms *en garde* on both sides of the brain and the mechanisms for reciprocal innervation and reciprocal inhibition constantly alerted for a refinement of movements unparalleled elsewhere. It is the ocular feedback innervation from each eye to both halves of the brain (more than proprioceptive feedback innervation from one hand to the opposite half of the brain) that makes the manipulations of the hand under the eye surgeon's operating microscope or under the scientist's micromanipulator possible. Fine hand movements need ocular control.[12]

How tightly knit the functional linkage is between medial rectus muscles, temporal retinas, and binocularity is best attested to by an analysis of convergence, a typically binocular oculorotary performance. Convergence (the simultaneous rolling of the two eyes toward each other) is initiated by the simultaneous displacement of fusable (identical or, at least, similar) images into the two temporal retinas, a displacement that, in its turn, stimulates simultaneous contraction of both medial rectus muscles (cf. Fig. 22). As one fixates the tip of a pencil and brings this fixation object gradually closer to his nose, the continuous displacement of the pencil's images from the foveas into the temporal retinas causes immediate consecutive adjustments (refixations) via the medial rectus muscles, the phenomenon called "convergence." (If the clinician lets a patient perform this "convergence exercise," he can follow the adjustment with the naked eye.) *Vice versa*, simultaneous stimulation of both *nasal* retinas by fusable images, *while the eyes are convergent*, permits relaxation of the contracted

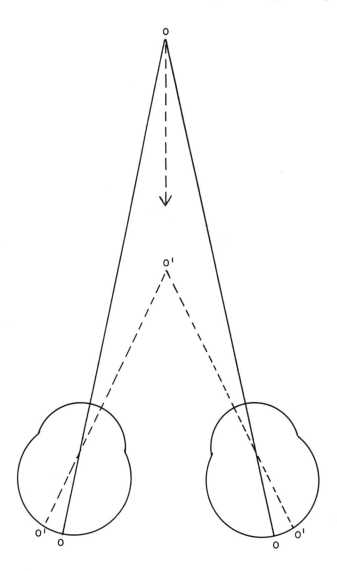

Fig. 22. Convergence. The eyes have their foveas *O* and *O* turned toward some object *O*. They fixate *O*. As soon as the object starts coming closer (in the direction indicated by *O'*) its images become displaced to the temporal half of each retina. This in turn stimulates the medial (inner) rectus muscles to contract. The eyes converge, and their gaze remains fixated on the object of attention in its new location.

medial rectus muscles and possibly even stimulates contraction of their antagonists, the lateral rectus muscles. As one fixates the pencil's tip and moves it away from his nose, the eyes will converge less and less. (There is no stimulation going to the temporal retinas.) And they would finally become parallel if the pencil could only reach "infinity." One cannot "diverge" eyes under physiologic conditions. The prime job of the nasal retinas and the lateral rectus muscles is not divergence but the coverage of the panorama. (One can, of course, make the eyes diverge slightly, say with appropriate prisms. But this is certainly not anything we want to analyze in this context.) The simple test I have just described, bringing some conspicuous small target (a small letter or picture is better than the tip of a pencil) closer and closer to the patient's nose is also a good test for dominance. The eyes converge as best they can. Finally, at the so-called near point of convergence, one eye "gives up" and straightens. It is generally the nondominant eye.

That ocular dominance is an operative entity, and not a spurious concept, is best attested to by clinical sighting tests. To convince ourselves, we can hand a child a toy gun and observe that from quite an early age the child will rather consistently aim the same eye at a target. An objectionable feature of this simple test is that hand dominance is too much involved. Sighting a target through a hole is preferable.

In my practice I use a cardboard from a laundered shirt (about 8 to 12 inches in size, with the long side horizontal) with a quarter-size hole cut in its center. I hand the cardboard to the patient; I make him hold it with two hands, in a symmetrical fashion, to neutralize the handedness factor as much as possible. I admonish the patient to hold his arms stretched out as far as he can reach and to grab the cardboard firmly (I make him perform a kind of Jendrássik maneuvre), all just to keep his mind off the performance of his eyes and to keep both hands equally busy. (The answers are most reliable if the patient does not even know what the test is all about.) I ask the patient to keep both eyes open, to elevate the cardboard to eye level, and to look through the hole at a light I hold in my hand or at a light at the other end of the room. (Sometimes I even pretend that I am doing a visual acuity test, letting the patient look at a single projected optotype letter on the opposite wall and then exchanging a larger letter for a smaller one as I repeat the test.) The patient, effectively, though inadvertently, excludes one eye from seeing the light or letter by holding the cardboard between the target and himself. He sights with what can be assumed to be his dominant eye; it certainly is his "sighting" eye. Letting a patient look into the barrel of a monocular microscope is an almost equally good test. (Boys love to look into my lensometer.) I might also mention in this context that most people will easily shut their nondominant eye, whereas it takes a conscious effort and some grimacing of face musculature to close the dominant eye. (I have mentioned that the convergence test also gives some indication.)

Sighting is, of course, a special kind of ocular activity. It is one of the few truly "aggressive" acts among all our visuomotor performances. (Early in this essay I referred to "aggressiveness" as the very circumstance which, through natural selection, made our race right-handed. It is probably this circumstance that made it right-eyed, at least right-sighting.) It is also a most ancient kind of a visuomotor performance. And finally it is a visuomotor performance that can be actuated with only *one* eye at a time. In the test described, the cardboard occludes one eye; in real life situations one inadvertently closes or in some other way excludes one eye while aiming a rifle using the other. Sighting is one of those instances in which early, primitive, uniocular, purely retinal directionalization along an ocular polar coordinate is still the most accurate and most effective mode of performance.[13] Binocularity would be a hindrance while aiming an arrow, not an advantage.[14]

I don't know, I confess, how much binocularity helps or hinders in throwing the javelin. A revolver, I am told, is fired with both eyes open. (I doubt the binocular character of the performance.) Patently, when sighting along an arrow or down a gun barrel, the performer returns to the Cyclops' space perception arrangement: the right half-retina of the sighting eye (whichever eye that is) reports to the right brain, and the left half-retina to the left brain. Theoretically, at least, it should make no difference in accurate aim of an arrow or a rifle whether one does it with the right eye or the left eye. The choice of eye is obviously *secondary* to the handedness-brainedness factor. It will be more convenient for a righthander to manipulate his visual world with the right eye (the right eye has a wider right visual field!) unless the performance of his two eyes is unequal. When visual acuities are unequal, he will generally sight with the eye with the better visual acuity. This obviously improves the quality of the aim. (I find that in the case of unequal astigmatism one almost invariably aims with the eye that has less astigmatism, even if clinically corrected visual acuity has resulted in equality of the two eyes.) In this case there might be a conflict between handedness and eyedness. One speaks of "crossed dominance," someone being, say, lefteyed, though right-handed. I remember one of my patients telling me the story of his tribulations in Army training, how desperately he tried to aim his gun with one eye while pulling the trigger with the opposite hand. But I also remember an affluent patient of mine, a passionate hunter, who, when a cataract started developing in one eye, had the butt of his gun so adjusted that he could sight with the other eye. (Unfortunately, I was not, at that time, interested in the problem and cannot remember details.) I think it would be useful if an Army health officer would study the details of eyedness-handedness in recruits beginning basic training. We might learn something about eyedness and crossed dominance.

In this conjunction, Benton's controlling eye test might be considered briefly. It is a binocular test; it endeavors to prove that when, in a small central area of the visual field, conditions for normal binocular fusional vision are suspended (and only under these conditions) one eye, which Benton calls the controlling eye, partly takes over and *hinders* the full perception performance of the other eye. Benton is right in not calling his test an ocular dominance test. It certainly has nothing to do with sighting performance; rather, it is a manifestation of contour inhibition, of a kind of rivalry between foreground and background, in this particular test, a contour in one eye, empty background in the other. It belongs in the sensory, not the motor, sphere of ocular performance, whereas our usual dominance tests have nothing to do with inhibition. I do not know what the statistical correlation is between eye dominance and Benton's phenomenon. I expect it must be rather high. Still for purposes of accuracy one has to decide whom to call, say, "righteyed." Is it the person whose right eye is his controlling eye in Benton's test, or the one whose right eye is his sighting eye? Hopefully, a consensus on this point will soon be reached. That I generally refer to the sighting eye as the dominant eye and call a person "righteyed" or "lefteyed" without further thought is probably just bad habit.

Benton's test will be better understood if we look at Fig. 23, a simplified diagram which serves demonstration purposes only. (In the actual test material, a stereogram arrangement, the patterns presented are somewhat more complex.) The essential features are ten dots (only five of the ten are shown) diminishing in size and presented only to one eye. Assume the left eye sees the pattern with dots; then the right eye sees those without dots. Assume that a patient sees eight of the ten dots (the dots are numbered) with the left eye *when his right eye is covered.* When the right eye is uncovered we will expect binocular ("fused") vision of all binocularly presented detail. What is of interest is the visibility of the dots under these conditions.

We would expect from the classic studies on contour (some are discussed in Linksz, 1952) that contour will always prevail, in rivalry, over noncontoured background, whereas Benton's phenomenon (and this is what is of interest) teaches us that this is not necessarily the case. It *can* happen that the left eye, when both eyes are open, sees only the first six of the presented dots, i.e., the background of what Benton calls the controlling eye suppresses the formation of minimum bulk contour[15] in the noncontrolling eye. A second stereogram, with dots presented only to the right eye, is needed to complete the test. Assume the following data in an individual case:

When dots are presented to the right eye only, "acuity" is

(a) monocular (only right eye open) 8
(b) binocular (both eyes open) 6

When dots are presented to the left eye only, "acuity" is

(a) monocularly (only left eye open) 8
(b) binocularly (both eyes open) 8

This establishes the left eye (in Benton's terminology) as the controlling eye. (In my clinical chart where space is at premium, I note:

Benton R 8 6!
 L 8 8

This describes the whole procedure and immediately tells me that it is the performance of the right eye that is inadequate.)

244

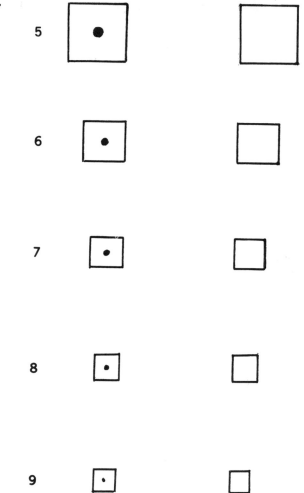

Fig. 23. Benton's test to find the controlling eye. The patterns are to be viewed in a stereoscope. Both eyes find identical squares presented to them. Their images fuse into a binocular but single percept. The dots of gradually diminishing size are seen only by the left eye. (Ten such sets of squares and dots are presented in the actual experiment. Here only dots 5 to 9 are shown. Also, the dots in the actual test material are much smaller.) First, we determine how many dots the left eye sees looking at the left-side pattern with the right eye closed or covered. Assume it sees eight out of the ten. When the right side pattern is *uncovered* and binocular fusional vision is established, two things can happen. If the number of dots seen by the left eye remains the same, the chances are that the left eye is the dominant or, as Benton calls it, the controlling eye. If the number of dots seen decreases to seven or six, the chances are that the right eye is dominant. (In the actual testing situation a second chart should also be used, with dots only on the right side.)

There is another item I feel I must mention in this connection. It is the phenomenon for which Ames et al. (1931) suggested the name "fixation disparity." It has since been extensively studied, especially by Ogle, and its name, now generally accepted (several others were proposed), describes it quite adequately. (An even more accurate though longer name would be "fixation with disparity" or still better, "binocular fixation with disparity.") It describes the fact that under certain experimental conditions which should permit what we call normal binocular vision, only one eye of a subject may turn its accurate fovea toward the object of fixation while the other eye assumes a slightly "disparate" position. (The condition is different from true squint: all other criteria of binocularity — fusion, "correspondence" of the retinas, stereopsis — are not materially impeded by its presence.)

Earlier I spoke of a "continuous undercurrent of monocular vision in spite of all the provisions for binocularity." While this is not an altogether normal occurrence, when it does occur fixation disparity permits us to observe both this undercurrent and the workings of ocular dominance, and this calls for a remark. An orthophoric subject (one who has no latent ocular muscular imbalance) generally shows no fixation disparity in our clinical tests, even if one or the other eye is strongly dominant: both of his eyes will be accurately fixated. However, if a patient has some kind of an ocular muscular imbalance ("heterophoria") and if this imbalance is permitted to make itself manifest by some kind of a binocularity-disturbing test arrangement (e.g., by looking into a stereoscope) then only one eye fixates accurately while the other deviates to the limit that maintenance of binocular single vision with fusion permits.[16] The eye that fixates accurately will be the dominant eye. The other eye will still partake in the binocular reception of impulses, but will do that less accurately. The subject will manifest the condition we have just defined as fixation disparity.

A stereogram arrangement by Hamburger (1960) permits testing for fixation disparity in a simple, yet reliable manner. The two patterns (Fig. 24) are presented in a stereoscope. Most details (the black triangles, the grid of squares, and the vertical row of three small dots on the right) are identical in the two halves of the stereogram. Each is seen by each eye, and they are fused (proper alignment and an existing faculty to binocular single vision being obvious prerequisites). The fused "image" serves as the *binocular* background. They don't show any disparity. Of the dots on the left side two are seen only by the right eye and one, the middle one, only by the left. My right eye is dominant, and at the same time I have some exophoria (my eyes tend to diverge). I see the left upper and the left lower dots well: they are steady and in the center of their respective square boxes. I see them through my right eye. At the same time, and in spite of all my fair binocular vision, the middle dot, seen only by my left eye, appears paler, is unsteady, and is displaced toward the right, indicating that I cannot actually accurately fixate a small target with my left eye as long as the right eye is open. I must look past it! My left eye turns outward, though only slightly, still permitting the fusion

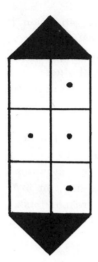

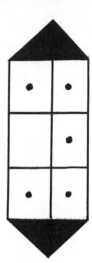

Fig. 24. Fixation disparity. Using a stereoscope, the right-hand pattern is viewed with the right eye and the left-hand pattern with the left eye. The "frames" are identical and, assuming normal or nearly normal binocular vision, the observer will see *one* frame binocularly. The same holds for the dots in the three right-hand boxes. They are seen by both eyes, and nothing stands in the way of fusion and binocular vision. However, the dots in the upper left and lower left box are seen only by the right eye, and the dot in the left center box is seen only by the left eye.

My right eye is dominant; there is an undercurrent of right-eye seeing, right-eye leading, to my binocularity. The dots seen only by my right eye appear to me as sharp, black, and steady, as the three binocularly seen dots do. My left eye is nondominant and has a tendency to outward rotation (exophoria). The dot seen by my left eye exclusively will appear fainter. It quivers slightly. It also appears slightly displaced from the exact center of the box, indicating that my left eye is turned slightly outward in spite of the lock effect of binocular single (fusional) vision. I actually fixate (if it can be called fixation) a "point" on the undifferentiated white background with my left fovea, a "point" somewhat to the left of the dot seen only by this eye, whereas the image of the dot falls on a retinal area slightly "off," temporal to, the true fovea. Since this latter area does not correspond (the technical phrase is "is disparate") to the fovea of my right eye, I see this dot in a different direction from that of the two dots localized in visual space by my right eye. *I fixate with disparity;* hence the term. If I close my right eye, the dot seen by my left eye suddenly becomes sharp, steady, and centered. When faced with the task of seeing "on its own" my nondominant eye performs quite well. Only when it has to apply itself in binocular vision does it become manifest that some stresses and strains have to be overcome to make binocularity feasible and that my left eye is the underdog.

In the actual testing situation the card should also be shown in an inverted manner, with the five dots to be seen by the left eye. In this case the left eye sees two quivering and slightly displaced dots.

of all fusable (= similar) details presented to both of my eyes. Thus, I not only fixate with disparity, I must be fusing with disparity. There is some constraint present when I use both eyes and some compromise. My left eye would "prefer" to turn further outward, but fusion (fusion of many strong contours) prevents it. (Fusion, binocular vision is not unalloyed bliss. Monocular vision is not an unmitigated calamity. As I said earlier, a crosseyed child has no eyestrain: a person with aniseikonia and compulsive binocular vision can be miserable.) The remarkable thing is that, as soon as I close my right dominant eye and look only with the left eye, that monocularly seen dot immediately becomes sharp, centered, and steady! (Note the similarity to Benton's phenomenon!)

Fixation disparity, when present, reveals which eye is dominant. It also reveals some of the characteristics of vision with the nondominant eye. Obviously, *ocular dominance preserves some of that steadiness of panoramic vision which binocularity cannot help disturbing to some extent.* Since the world as seen binocularly cannot ever offer absolutely identical patterns to both eyes (this can only be achieved in a well-controlled laboratory experiment), convergence on any real target details in our surround can never be as steady as our diagrams of convergence make us believe. Images of "real" objects received by the two eyes cannot help being disparate per se, even if our clinical tests (always artificial) show "perfect balance" and no fixation disparity. *We have to close one eye (the nondominant one) and revert to the maximum security and steadiness of cyclopean vision, of the Cyclops' vision, when aiming a gun becomes a matter of life and death.*

Fixation disparity is, by necessity, always tested for by some deliberate disruption of binocular vision, however slight. All our tests of binocular vision and stereopsis cause — this is inevitable — some disruption of (or encroachment on) the natural conditions of vision.

Fixation disparity reveals that fusion is under duress. Confuse a patient who is exophoric by shining a rather bright light into his eyes. He will inadvertently close the nondominant eye, which, by the way, is another way of testing for ocular dominance.

I do not believe that the preferred hand is the sole determinant of eyedness, though I think that handedness is a prime determinant. Eyedness might even be changeable. But I am certainly not in accord with authorities like Parson (1924) who believe that eyedness is primary to handedness. I cannot altogether believe in the devastating significance of reading difficulties attributed to lefteyedness. Neither have I found in my clinical practice any convincing evidence that so-called mixed dominance is a frequent cause or even a collateral of reading retardation. Though I do not have any experience in the matter, I cannot believe that if handedness is changed to conform with eyedness reading performance will materially improve. Of course, all these ideas, opinions, statements, results are in a kind of flux nowadays. We will have to wait until unbiased research produces some unbiased answers.

NOTES

[1]However restricted it is, the total visual field of the two eyes can still be called a "panorama," and it is almost needless to remind the reader that its right and left half meet on a vertical line, not at a point. Point O is merely a point on the horizontal cross section through the visual field which is all that can be indicated in this type of diagram. What we must understand is that each half of the panorama covers the opposite half of the visual cortex; together they provide a cyclopean "map" of the total panorama. It should be added that the two brain halves are also separated by a vertical divider: a vertical groove cuts the brain (at least the crown of the brain) into a right hemisphere and a left hemisphere.

[2]In contradistinction to the bird of prey we have only one set of foveas.

[3]Walls (1963) suggested a simple experiment: "Prolong" your nose by placing one of your hands vertically snug against your nose and look straight ahead. You prevent the temporal half-retina of your left eye from covering the right visual field and the temporal half-retina of your right eye from covering the left visual field. Still, you are visually aware of the totality of your panorama. There is no break. Nothing is missing. For orientation in space we don't need our temporal half-retinas.

[4]As a matter of fact, newer studies (see Geschwind, 1972) indicate definite asymmetry between the two temporal lobes, a greater "bulk" on the left side in the majority of cases.

[5]Clinicians call the conjugated rotation of the two eyes in the same direction an ocular "version," dextroversion, levoversion, etc.

[6]The word for yoke is *iugum* in Latin — hence the term "conjugated" given in the previous footnote.

[7]In a precious little volume, *Goethe on Nature and Science*, Sir Charles Sherrington (1942) writes: "He seems sometimes, as we listen to him, to be looking over the shoulder of a creative Being, and entranced by watching her amid her work."

[8]Each superior-oblique eye rotator muscle also has its separate nerve trunk and its nucleus. To consider the reasons for this would lead us too far from our present subject of inquiry.

[9]In contradistinction to the term "version," clinicians use the term "vergence" to cover such adjustments for fusion.

[10]See the impact of, say, the right eye on the visual context in Fig. 21.

[11]This is true even when only one eye is seeing. When both eyes are open the quality of a stereopsis is added, that superb refinement of binocular near vision which I cannot discuss here. (See Linksz, 1952 for an analysis of stereopsis.)

[12]Music making is an obvious exception. The performance of a blind pianist may be supreme. His motor orientation within his instrument's confines (but only within his instrument's confines) works on a purely aural feedback. He hears the notes as he hits the keys. The performance of a blind typist is actually more amazing. His orientation is purely by bodyschema. He has learned how far he has to reach to hit a certain key. But he has no way to ascertain if he has hit the right one. He lacks any feedback information about the performance of his hands.

[13]In principle it could be any coordinate. We could align the barrel of a gun with any retinal point as long as that point is covered by the image of our target (is aligned with the target). That we first bring the target's image upon the best-seeing area (the fovea) of our sighting eye is a matter of convenience and efficiency, not a theoretical necessity.

[14]Galathea was seemingly not too far off the mark when she commented on her suitor's superior visual performance. He was a warrior, not a craftsman.

[15]Benton's phenomenon is observable only with small objects, like small black dots on a white background near the threshold of visibility. Large contours, redoubled contours, always "prevail" over any contourless unstructured background.

[16]According to data by Jampolsky et al. (1957) the probability that a subject will have considerable fixation disparity is greater if the tendency of his eyes is to turn toward each other ("esophoria"). In this case, the disparate image falls on the nasal retina of the less accurately aligned eye. It seems that even in matters of fixation disparity nasal and temporal retina halves behave differently.

REFERENCES

Ames, A., Jr., Gliddon, G. H., and Ogle, K. N. Corresponding retinal points, the horopter and size and shape of ocular images. J. Opt. Soc. Am. 22:665, 1932.

Ariens Kappers, C. U. On structural laws in the nervous system: the principles of neurobiotaxis. Brain 44:125, 1921.

Benton, C. J. Management of dyslexias associated with binocular control abnormalities. In Keeney, A. H., and Keeney, V. T., Eds. Dyslexia. St. Louis, Mosby, 1968.

Bolinger, D. Aspects of Language. Harcourt, New York, 1968.

Buswell, G. T. Suppl. Educ. Monogr. 21, 1922. Quoted from Wadsworth, 1938.

Cajal, S. R. Histologie du système nerveux de l'homme et des vertébrés. Paris, Maloine, 1911.

Chall, J. S. Learning to Read: The Great Debate. New York, McGraw-Hill, 1967.

Dejerine, J. Sur un cas de cécité verbale avec agraphie, suivi d'autopsie. C. R. Soc. Biol. (Paris) iii:197, 1891.

Dejerine, J. Contribution a l'étude anatomopathologique et clinique des différentes variétés de cécité verbale. C. R. Soc. Biol. (Paris) iv:61, 1892.

Diringer, D. Writing. New York, Praeger, 1962.

Flesch, R. Why Johnny Can't Read. New York, Harper, 1955.

Flom, M. C., Heath, G. G., and Takahashi, E. Contour interaction and visual resolution: contralateral effects. Science 142:979, 1963.

Flom, M. C., Weymouth, F. W., and Kaneman, D. Visual resolution and contour interaction. J. Opt. Soc. Am. 53:1026, 1963.

Fremantle, A. The Age of Belief. New York, Mentor (New American Library), 1955.

Freud, S. Zur Auffassung der Aphasien. Vienna, Deuticke, 1891.

Gelb, I. J. A Study in Writing. Chicago, University of Chicago Press, 1963.

Geschwind, N. Language and the brain. Sci. Am. 226/4:76 (April), 1972.

Goethe, J. W. von.* Die Natur. J. von Tiefurt, 32 Stück, 1782.

Goldberg, H. K. Vision, perception and related facts in dyslexia. In Keeney and Keeney, Eds., Dyslexia. St. Louis, Mosby, 1968.

Goodglass, H., and Quadfasel, F. A. Language laterality in left-handed aphasics. Brain 77:521, 1954.

Hamburger, F. A. Stellungsanomalien. in Velhagen, K., Ed., Der Augenarzt. Stuttgart, Thieme, 1960, p. 817.

Jackson, J. Hughlings. Evolution and dissolution of the Nervous system. In Taylor, J., Ed. Selected Writings of John Hughlings Jackson, Vol. 2. New York, Basic Books, 1958.

Jampolsky, A., Flom, M. C., and Fried, A. N. Fixation disparity in relation to heterophoria. Am. J. Ophthalmol. 43:1, 1957.

Kalmus, H. Diagnosis and Genetics of Defective Colour Vision. Oxford, Pergamon, 1965.

Kalmus, H. Genetics. New York, Doubleday, 1964.

Keeney, A. H., and Keeney, V. T., Eds. Dyslexia. St. Louis, Mosby, 1968.

Keeney, A. H.: Case studies in dyslexia. Trans. Am. Ophthalmol. Soc. 67:68, 1969.

Kolers, P. A. Bilingualism and information processing. Sci. Am. 218/3:78 (March), 1968.

Linksz, A. An ophthalmologist looks at art and artists. Proc. Am.-Hungar. Med. Assoc. 1:60, 1965.

Linksz, A. Physiology of the Eye, Vol. II, Vision. New York, Grune & Stratton, 1952.

Moorhouse, A. C. The Triumph of the Alphabet. New York, Schuman, 1953.

Orton, S. T. Reading, Writing, and Speech Problems in Children. New York, Norton, 1937.

Parson, B. S. Lefthandedness. New York, Macmillan, 1924.

Quadfasel, F. A., and Goodglass, H. Specific reading disability and other specific disabilities. J. Learning Disabilities 1:590, 1968.

Rosner, S. L. Dyslexia: a problem in definition. Am. Orthopt. J. 18:94, 1968.

*Modern Goethe scholars attribute this famous paper (reading of which made Freud decide to study medicine) to one of Goethe's young friends, a member of the circle of Goethe's friends and patrons. (Personal communication of the late Professor Johannes Urzidil, poet and Goethe scholar.)

Sherrington, C. Goethe on Nature and on Science. Cambridge, Cambridge University Press, 1949.

Uexküll, J. von, and Kriszat, G. Streifzüge durch die Umwelten von Tieren und Menschen. Berlin, Springer, 1934.

Walls, G. L. The Vertebrate Eye and Its Adaptive Radiation. New York, Hafner, 1963.

Wertheimer, M. Untersuchungen uben dar Sehen von Bewegungen. Z. Psychol. 161:265, 1912.

Whorf, B. L., Carroll, J. B., Eds. In Language, Thought, and Reality, Cambridge, Mass., MIT, 1956.

Wölfflin, H. Classic Art. London, Phaidon, 1952.

Woodworth, R. S. Experimental Psychology. New York, Holt, 1938.

Abducens. The sixth of the twelve pairs of so-called cranial nerves whose function is innervation of the lateral rectus muscles.

Afferent. Carrying neural messages from the periphery toward the brain. (See *Efferent.*)

Alexia. Loss of previously acquired ability to read.

Algorithm. The art of calculating by means of nine figures and zero.

Alveolar. Pertaining to the parts of the jaws where the sockets (alveolae) of the teeth are situated; specifically, designation of the consonant sounds produced by pressing the tongue against these parts (phoneticists call /d/ a "voiced" and /t/ a "voiceless" alveolar stop).

Amblyopia. Poor vision with no physical reason in evidence; specifically, no apparent change in ocular structures.

Aniseikonia (an = no, is = equal, eikon = image, ia = condition). Condition in which the images formed in the two eyes do not match.

Aspirate. A consonant produced by breathing (e.g., the sound /h/).

Astigmia, astigmatism. Condition in which rays from object point fail to come to point focus (a = no, stigma = point); specifically, condition in which rays of light from visible object point fail to come to point focus within the optics of the eye.

Binocular (single) vision. Single vision brought about by blending ("fusion") of the views presented to the two eyes.

Boustrophedon. Writing alternating lines in opposite directions.

Broca's area. An area in the (left) frontal lobe that controls articulate speech (not the individual muscles involved).

Caudal. Direction toward "tail" (downward).

Cognate. Having same or similar origin.

Convergence. Simultaneous turn of both eyes inward (nasalward), presumably to fixate (bifixate and fuse) near object of regard.

Coronal. See *Cranial.*

Cranial. Direction toward the brain (upward) (also called *coronal*).

Cyclops (Cyclopean). A giant of Greek mythology having but one eye.

Dextroversion (levoversion). Turning of the eye to the right (left).

253

Diacritical mark (sign). A sign attached to a letter to distinguish it from another letter. (See *Umlaut.*)

Digraph. A group of two vowels or (rarely) consonants representing a single speech sound (in CHAIR, the first two letters form a consonant digraph, and the next two letters a vowel digraph modulated by the final R).

Diphthong. Continuous change of vowel sound from one into another within a single syllable (e.g., in HOUSE).

Diplopia. Double vision — seeing two objects where there is only one to be seen.

Dyslexia (as defined in the context of this volume). Difficulty in reading, in acquiring the reading skill.

Efferent. Carrying neural messages from the brain toward the periphery. (See *Afferent.*)

Emmetropia ("normal" refraction). Condition in which rays from distant visible objects gather in a "point" on retina.

Extraocular muscles. See *Rectus muscles, Oblique muscles.*

Fovea ("pit"). A restricted retinal region whose sensory discriminative capacity is maximal.

Fusion, binocular fusion. The formation of a unitary percept from visual stimuli reaching both eyes.

Grapheme. The letters that represent one phoneme. (See *Phoneme.*)

Hemianopia. Lack of sight in one-half of the visual field. *Binasal hemianopia.* Lack of sight in both nasal visual fields. *Bitemporal hemianopia.* Lack of sight in both temporal visual fields.

Heterophoria. Tendency of eyes to dissociate, loss of parallel stance of eyes when fusion *(q.v.)* is prevented; specifically, *exophoria* (esophoria), tendency of eyes to diverge (converge) when fusion is prevented; *hyper-* or *hypophoria,* tendency of one eye to move upward (the other eye to move downward) when fusion is prevented. (See also *Ocular muscular imbalance.*)

Heterotropia. Esotropia, Condition in which one eye is turned inward (nasally, toward the nose) in excess of what is normal, while the other eye is presumably straight. *Exotropia,* condition in which one eye is turned outward (laterally, toward the temple) while the other eye is presumably straight.

Homograph. One, two, or more words spelled alike but different in meaning.

Homophone. One, two, or more words pronounced alike but different in meaning (and spelling).

Hypermetropia (so-called farsightedness). Condition in which rays from distant visible object fail to gather (come into focus) on retina; condition in which convex ("plus") lenses are needed for correction.

Ideogram. A conventionalized symbol that symbolizes a thing or idea (but not necessarily the same spoken word).

Lobe. A major division of the brain (e.g., *temporal lobe*, the one located near the "temple").

Morpheme. A meaningful linguistic unit that contains no meaningful smaller parts (e.g., HAT).

Myopia (so-called nearsightedness). Condition in which rays from distant visible object come to focus *in front* of retina; condition in which concave ("minus") lenses are needed for correction.

Nasal (temporal). Direction toward the nose (temple), location nearer nose (temple).

Nystagmus. Rapid involuntary oscillation of the eyes.

Oblique muscles. Two pairs of extraocular muscles (involved in some more complex ocular rotations not discussed in this text).

Ocular (binocular) muscular imbalance. Difficulty of directing both eyes at the same object point. (See *Heterophoria*.)

Oculomotorius. The name of the third pair of cranial nerves. (They marshal four of the six pairs of eye muscles.)

Ontogenetic. See *Phylogenetic*.

Parturition. Childbirth, delivery.

Phoneme. Smallest unit of speech that distinguishes one utterance from another (the /p/ in *pin*, the /f/ in *fin* are two different phonemes).

Phonogram. A written (printed) symbol that represents a phoneme, syllable, or word.

Phylogenetic. Pertaining to the racial history of an organism, as distinguished from *ontogenetic*, pertaining to the development of the individual organism.

Pyramidal tract. One of the columns of motor nerve fibers that, on their way toward the spinal chord, cross the midline.

Ray. The imaginary trajectory of a particle of light.

Rectus muscles. Four pairs of extraocular muscles to move the eyes in unison (roughly), up, down, right, or left, respectively.

Refraction. Deflection of rays at the boundary between two transparent media, specifically, the deflection of rays falling on the eye.

Refraction error, refractive error, ametropia. (See *Hypermetropia, Myopia, Astigmatism*.)

Retina. The inner lining of the eyeballs in which occurs the transformation of the optical image into physiologic process.

Strabismus, squint. See *Heterotropia*.

Stereopsis. Capacity of depth perception with two eyes receiving essentially equal but horizontally slightly disparate images.

Strephosymbolia (literally, twisted symbols). Condition of confused dominance of the cerebral hemispheres.

Third nerve. See *Oculomotorius*.

Umlaut. Shift of vowel sound from "back" (or "low") to "front" (or "high") to change a word's grammatical standing (e.g., LOUSE/ LICE); in German, placing a diacritical mark /../ on top of a "back" (or "low") vowel to effect this change (e.g., LAUS/ LÄUSE).

Vergence. Adaptive rotation of the eyes to safeguard binocular foveal vision. (See *Convergence*.)

Version. Conjugated rotation of the two eyes in the same direction.

Wernicke's area. Coordinating "center" in the temporal lobe (of the left brain), stationed between the auditory and visual receiving stations and Broca's area *(q.v.)*.